Parkinson's Disease

An In-depth
Metabolic Guide

Ray Griffiths MSc

© 2019 Ray Griffiths

First edition: June 2019

All rights reserved. No part of this publication may be reproduced, distributed, or transmitted in any form or by any means, including photocopying, recording, or other electronic or mechanical methods, without the prior written permission of the publisher, except in the case of brief quotations embodied in critical reviews and certain other non-commercial uses permitted by copyright law. For permission requests, write to the publisher at the email address below.

raybakes@yahoo.com

ISBN: 978-1-07-382485-4

Cover design and typesetting:
David Siddall Multimedia, Monmouth, UK
www.davidsiddall.com

*To Karen, Brian, Catherine, Genevieve,
Alex, Tim, Xavier, Richard and Kate*

By the same author:

Mitochondria in Health and Disease

Depression: The Mind-Body Diet and Lifestyle Connection

Contents

Introduction vii

    Dopamine Metabolism 1

    Dopamine Synthesis 5

    L-DOPA, Dopamine and Parkinson's Disease 6

    Nutrition, L-DOPA and Dopamine 8

    Misfolded Proteins – α-Synuclein 10

    Lysosomal α-Synuclein Degradation 14

    Mitochondria and Parkinson's Disease 17

    α-Synuclein and Fatigue 21

    The Endoplasmic Reticulum 23

    The Benzene Ring, Health and Disease 25

    Fatty Acids. A New Understanding 29

    Cholesterol and Parkinson's Disease.
    Contradictory Evidence 35

    Lipid Rafts 37

    The Light Side of Oestrogen and Parkinson's
    Disease 40

    The Dark Side of Oestrogen and Dopamine
    Metabolites 41

    Microglia 46

    Blood-Brain Barrier and Neurovascular Unit 51

    The Glymphatic System 57

    Metals and Ions and Neurotoxicity 58

    Heat-shock Proteins and Chaperones 62

    Type 2 Diabetes and the Risk of Parkinson's
    Disease 65

    The Cytoskeleton and Neurodegeneration 68

    Psychological Stress 70

    L-DOPA-induced Dyskinesias (LIDs) 71

Aromatic L-amino Acid Decarboxylase (AADC) Inhibitors........73
Biomarkers for Parkinson's Disease..75
Tyrosine Kinase Inhibition 76
Uric Acid 78
Ketogenic Diet...80
Can Nutritional Intervention Help Repair Dopaminergic Synapses?..83
Bibliography 87
Further reading... 120
Index 121

Introduction

Over the last ten years there has been a quantum leap in our understanding of the mechanisms which drive neurodegeneration and Parkinson's disease. Frustratingly, this new research has not yet managed to infiltrate mainstream medical and public perceptions of the disease, where Parkinson's disease is still seen purely as a dopamine deficiency condition. It is hoped that this book will give the reader an accessible insight into these exciting new discoveries.

Although some of the material is quite technical, each aspect of Parkinson's disease has been broken down into short manageable chapters. This concise presentation will enable the reader to dip in and out of the text where necessary.

The new research includes:

The Catecholaldehyde hypothesis – DOPAL, the toxic aldehyde metabolite of dopamine which, if produced in excess, or not detoxified sufficiently, may lead to neurodegeneration. Please see the chapter **Dopamine Metabolism** for more details.

The Braak hypothesis – The misfolded protein α-synuclein may be present in gut or olfactory nerves before appearing in dopaminergic neurons. Misfolded protein aggregates or Lewy bodies may seed themselves through the nervous system over time. These proteins may eventually reach a part of the brain called the substantia nigra and play a major role in Parkinson's disease pathology. The chapter **Misfolded Proteins – α-Synuclein** has further information on the Braak hypothesis.

The MAM hypothesis – The mitochondria-associated ER membrane (MAM) implicates many of the main protagonists now associated with Parkinson's disease. Many of the brain areas affected by Parkinson's disease are dependent on correct MAM function. The chapters **The Endoplasmic Reticulum** and **Lipid Rafts** have more information regarding the MAM hypothesis.

The Autophagy-Lysosome Pathway (ALP) – The ALP is an important cellular 'waste bin' and the failure of this pathway can lead to a neuron malfunctioning due to an excessive accumulation of cellular waste. The chapter **Lysosomal α-Synuclein Degradation** expands on how the ALP is implicated in Parkinson's disease.

Lipid rafts – These floating 'fatty islands' within membranes act like signalling 'junction boxes' for much of the immune system. By manipulating dietary and endogenous fats, profound changes can be effected throughout the nervous and immune systems. Please refer to the chapter **Lipid Rafts**.

Microglial activation – Chronic activation of microglia, the resident immune cells of the central nervous system (CNS), may lead to neuroinflammatory conditions like Parkinson's disease. Microglia are discussed in the chapter **Microglia** and also throughout the rest of the book.

The Glymphatic system – Clearance of waste products and misfolded proteins from the brain via the glymphatic system is vital to help protect against neurodegenerative conditions such as Parkinson's and Alzheimer's diseases. Please refer to the chapter **The Glymphatic System**.

Metabolic syndrome – Type 2 diabetes, insulin resistance and metabolic syndrome all have associations with neurodegeneration and Parkinson's disease via multiple mechanisms. Degenerative diseases can no longer be viewed as isolated conditions; much of the pathology which drives metabolic syndrome will also be implicated in neurodegenerative disease. Please read the chapter **Type 2 Diabetes and the Risk of Parkinson's Disease** for further information.

What is becoming clear is that Parkinson's disease is a complex multifactorial disease where many ill-functioning aspects of health intersect to cause a failure of the dopaminergic system. To seek a singular cause amongst such complexity is likely to be futile but, hopefully, the themes in this book may help the reader to see emergent patterns of the disease. Each Parkinson's disease patient is likely to display their own patterns and vulnerabilities which have become their own unique triggers for the disease.

At present, even with all the knowledge we have of the many mechanisms behind Parkinson's disease, we can still at best only slow progression of the disease. There is still so much more that needs to be learnt and discovered before major inroads can be made into changing the course of Parkinson's disease in patients.

Prevention is clearly still the best the best course of action for Parkinson's disease. Around 95% of the disease is due to poor diet and lifestyle choices, meaning that there is so much individuals can do to protect themselves. It may be stating the obvious but addressing poor diet, stress, constipation, lack of exercise and insulin resistance/obesity will give many of us a head start in avoiding this all too common degenerative disease.

Dopamine Metabolism

The key features of Parkinson's disease were originally described by James Parkinson in his 1817 paper "Essay on the Shaking Palsy". Parkinson's disease is the second most common neurodegenerative disease after Alzheimer's disease and affects 1% of the population over 65 (Gibrat et al. 2009).

Parkinson's disease is caused by the loss of dopaminergic neurons in the *substantia nigra pars compacta*, a region located in the mid-brain, which forms part of the basal ganglia. Axons of dopaminergic neurons from the *substantia nigra pars compacta* extend into the striatum, forming the nigrostriatal pathway, the route which supplies dopamine to the striatum (Dauer & Przedborski 2003).

Symptoms of Parkinson's disease occur when around 60% of dopaminergic neurons are lost (Dauer & Przedborski 2003). Depletion of nigrostriatal dopamine in the basal ganglia leads to the characteristic slowness of movement called akinesia and bradykinesia. These symptoms occur alongside tremor, rigidity and altered gait (Thomas 2009).

Dopamine metabolism

Dopamine (DA) is synthesised from L-DOPA within the cytosol of a dopaminergic neuron. Dopamine is subsequently sequestered into a synaptic vesicle by vesicular monoamine transporter 2 (VMAT2). When a dopaminergic neuron is activated, the vesicle then releases dopamine into the synapse. Re-uptake of dopamine occurs via the dopamine transporter (DAT), and dopamine is then re-sequestered into a vesicle by VMAT2 (Meiser et al. 2013).

Dopamine is an unstable compound in the cytosol and may undergo autoxidation, forming dopamine quinones, hydrogen peroxide and superoxide (Dauer & Przedborski 2003).

Dopamine quinones may inhibit complex I of the mitochondrial electron transport chain, leading to reductions in ATP synthesis and energy (Jana et al. 2011). Tyrosine hydroxylase (the rate-limiting enzyme of dopamine synthesis) can have its normal activity inhibited by dopamine quinones, resulting in increased ROS synthesis by the enzyme (Kuhn et al. 1999).

Dopamine tends to remain stable when sequestered into the lower pH (increased acidity) and MAO-free environment of the vesicle (Lotharius & Brundin 2002). However, neurotoxins such as 1-methyl-4-phenylpyridinium (MPP$^+$), amphetamine, rotenone and α-synuclein may slow sequestering of dopamine into the vesicle, or trigger leakage of dopamine back into the cytosol. The negative effects of these toxic compounds will therefore mean that dopamine will remain in the harsh environment of the cytosol too long, increasing chances of dopamine oxidation neuronal damage (Goldstein et al. 2013).

Dopamine – the biochemistry

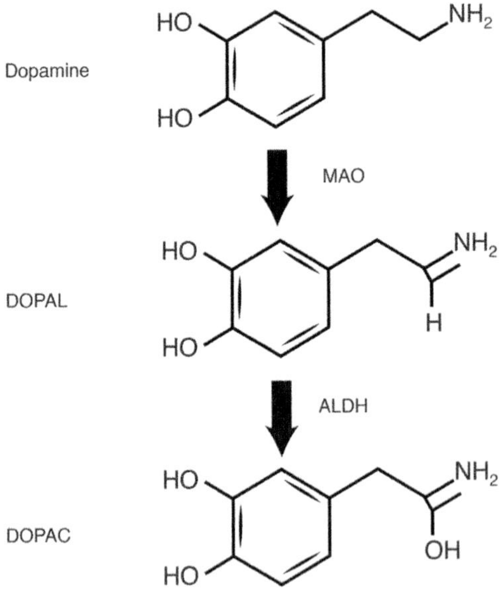

Dopamine

DOPAL

DOPAC

Dopamine is normally degraded by the enzyme monoamine oxidase (MAO). This first step of dopamine degradation produces the potentially toxic by-products hydrogen peroxide, ammonia and DOPAL (3,4-dihydroxyphenylacetaldehyde), an aldehyde estimated to be 1000 more toxic than dopamine (Burke 2003).

The second step clears DOPAL via the enzyme aldehyde dehydrogenase (ALDH) to produce a more benign by-product DOPAC. In ageing and Parkinson's disease there tends to be an increase in MAO activity and a decrease in ALDH, leading to higher amounts of DOPAL, alongside its potential toxicity.

The presence of DOPAL in the cytosol can lead to increased production of lipid peroxides such as 4-hydroxynonenal (4HNE), an inhibitor of ALDH (Goldstein et al. 2013). Therefore, DOPAL can create a cellular environment which inhibits its own detoxification, effectively leading to an amplification of its toxicity.

The catecholaldehyde hypothesis

In Parkinson's disease patients, there is a five-fold increase in toxic DOPAL levels in the putamen of the brain. This increase is thought to be due to an estimated 90% reduction in VMAT2 activity and a 70% reduction in ALDH activity. In normal dopaminergic neurons, 90% of cytosolic dopamine is sequestered into vesicles by VMAT2, thereby protecting the neuron from excessive DOPAL toxicity (Goldstein et al. 2013); (Eisenhofer et al. 2004).

Considering the potential toxicity of increased cytosolic DOPAL from L-DOPA therapy, several studies, surprisingly, claim to not have found any negative effects from L-DOPA therapy (Rajput et al. 1997); (Rajput 2001).

The drugs selegiline and rasagiline are MAO inhibitors, which not only increase the availability of dopamine, but may also modulate the degradation of dopamine, to help reduce the rapid increases in DOPAL after L-DOPA therapy.

Rasagiline is considered to be a superior and safer MAO-inhibitor to selegiline, since selegiline produces potentially toxic amphetamine compounds during its metabolism (McCormack 2014). In addition, selegiline has been linked with sleep disturbance in Parkinson's disease patients (Albers et al. 2017).

Some researchers have named the combined failure of MAO, ALDH, DAT and VMAT2 (to allow the safe activity and sequestration of dopamine) the 'catecholaldehyde hypothesis' (Goldstein et al. 2013).

Nutrition and Dopamine metabolism
MAO-inhibition

Curcumin, luteolin, quercetin, ursolic acid, rutin, catechin and berry anthocyanins are compounds in plants which all have some degree of MAO-inhibitory activity (Carradori et al. 2014); (Dreiseitel et al. 2009).

Rasagiline and selegiline tend to inhibit MAO to a greater extent and for a longer duration than plant compounds. For example, rasagiline can continue to inhibit 40% of MAO in the brain, even 13 days after the last dose (Youdim et al. 2001).

Phenolic compounds from plants of the mint family have both MAO-inhibitory and ALDH-stimulating activity, and can help protect against α-synuclein aggregation, one of the signature pathologies in Parkinson's disease (Mazzio et al. 2013); (Caruana et al. 2011).

In animal models, it has been found that lower dietary and brain levels of omega-3 fatty acids, particularly DHA, can lead to increases in MAO-B activity, with concomitant decreases in dopamine in some regions of the brain. Furthermore, omega-3 deficiency resulted in reduced VMAT2 function, leading to depletion of dopamine in the storage vesicles (Müller et al. 2014).

Additional protective dietary compounds for dopamine metabolism

Berberine, isolated from the fruit of the shrub barberry (*Berberis vulgaris L.*) has been found to prevent loss of dopaminergic neurons. In animal models berberine prevented neuronal damage – if these results translate to human patients, berberine could possibly alleviate memory and motor impairment in Parkinson's disease patients (Kim et al. 2014).

ALDH-2 is the mitochondrial isoform of ALDH. ALDH-2 contains redox sensitive thiol groups which may deactivate the enzyme in the presence of excessive ROS. This may explain some of the beneficial actions of reducing agents (antioxidants) in Parkinson's disease (Wenzel et al. 2007).

ALDH activity has been shown to be supported by the nutraceuticals taurine, lipoic acid and pantethine (McCarty 2013). The green algae chlorella has been found to be supportive of ALDH activity in laboratory animals (Nakashima et al. 2014).

Dopamine Synthesis

It is the loss of dopaminergic neurons and the associated dopamine synthesis which leads to the characteristic motor symptoms and tremor seen in Parkinson's disease.

The biochemical journey for this neurotransmitter starts with dietary protein and amino acids, and then on to L-DOPA (L-3,4-dihydroxyphenylalanine), to cross the blood-brain barrier. Dopamine is synthesised from L-DOPA within dopaminergic neurons.

Dopamine, along with noradrenaline (norepinephrine) and adrenaline (epinephrine) are all from a family of compounds called catecholamines. Dopamine is an intermediate in adrenaline and noradrenaline synthesis, as well as a neurotransmitter in its own right. Catecholamines, including dopamine, are synthesised from the amino acids phenylalanine and tyrosine.

The amino acid tyrosine undergoes hydroxylation via the enzyme tyrosine hydroxylase, forming the dopamine precursor L-DOPA. Dopamine is in turn the product of the action of the enzyme aromatic amino acid decarboxylase (AADC) on L-DOPA (Berry & Boulton 2013).

Dopamine is the most prevalent catecholamine in the central nervous system where it is in control of locomotor activity, cognition, emotion, positive reinforcement, food intake, and endocrine regulation.

Outside the central nervous system, dopamine has functions associated with gastrointestinal motility, vascular tone, kidney, cardiovascular and hormone regulation.

In addition to Parkinson's disease, dysregulation of dopamine has been associated with schizophrenia, hyperprolactinaemia, Tourette's syndrome and ADHD (Missale et al. 1998); (Swanson et al. 2000).

L-DOPA, Dopamine and Parkinson's Disease

Researchers in the early 1960s discovered that Parkinson's disease was associated with failures in the dopaminergic system, and they found reduced levels of dopamine in the brains of patients (Berry & Boulton 2013). This discovery led to the use of L-DOPA (L-3,4-dihydroxyphenylalanine) as a drug to help with Parkinson's disease symptoms. L-DOPA/levodopa has been viewed as the 'gold standard' of Parkinson's disease care since its development, although it is not thought to significantly alter the course of the disease.

Decarboxylase inhibitors – helping L-DOPA to cross the blood-brain barrier

Dopamine is unable to cross the blood-brain barrier, but its precursor L-DOPA readily crosses the blood-brain barrier. Since the mid-1970s, L-DOPA/levodopa has been formulated with the aromatic amino acid decarboxylase inhibitors carbidopa and benserazide. Both these inhibitors help prevent the peripheral conversion of L-DOPA to dopamine (Meiser et al. 2013).

The combination of L-DOPA/levodopa and decarboxylase inhibitor leads to greater efficacy of the drug, with substantially more L-DOPA/levodopa reaching target neurons. Therefore, less of the drug can be prescribed, resulting in fewer side effects.

Issues with tyrosine hydroxylase, the rate-limiting enzyme for dopamine synthesis

Tyrosine hydroxylase (TH) is the rate-limiting enzyme for dopamine synthesis. TH is dependent on iron and the co-factor biopterin. When active, TH produces reactive oxygen species (which can be damaging to dopaminergic neurons). In some neurons, ageing may lead to a decrease in TH activity, but in others, loss of dopamine may lead to reduced negative feedback to the enzyme, with a consequent increase in ROS production.

L-DOPA/levodopa can have an antioxidant effect by providing negative feedback to TH, thereby lessening reactive oxygen species generation (Adams et al. 1997). Alternatively, L-DOPA/levodopa can increase neuronal toxicity by raising levels of the neurotoxic aldehyde DOPAL.

Tyrosine hydroxylase (TH) itself can be damaged by oxidised dopamine and L-DOPA. This results in TH being converted to a ROS-generating, redox-cycling quinoprotein called 'quinotyrosine hydroxylase' (Kuhn et al. 1999).

Nutrition, L-DOPA and Dopamine

L-DOPA and dopamine are directly derived from the dietary amino acids phenylalanine and tyrosine. There are several other compounds, linked to diet and nutrition, which can also influence and enhance dopamine synthesis. Human metabolism is a web of biochemistry, profoundly influenced by, and dependent on, diet and nutrition.

Biopterin

Biopterin is an essential co-factor for the enzyme tyrosine hydroxylase, but can also undergo autoxidation, leading to the generation of superoxide, hydrogen peroxide and hydroxyl radicals (Adams et al. 1997).

Normally, supplementation of the amino acid tyrosine will lead to a threefold to sevenfold increase in serum biopterin. However, serum biopterin in Parkinson's disease patients is much reduced.

In Parkinson's disease patients, tyrosine supplementation will produce less than a twofold increase in biopterin (Yamaguchi et al. 1983). Biopterin is required, in its active form, to maintain tyrosine hydroxylase activity. Glutathione, ascorbate and NADH (nicotinamide adenine dinucleotide) can all help to keep the enzyme in its active form (Wei et al. 2003).

Vitamin B6

The conversion of L-DOPA to dopamine requires the vitamin-B6-dependent enzyme amino acid decarboxylase (AADC). Carbidopa and benserazide are included in L-DOPA medication to inhibit AADC.

Inhibiting AADC halts the peripheral conversion of L-DOPA to dopamine, before L-DOPA can cross the blood-brain barrier. This has the effect of increasing the amount of L-DOPA crossing the blood-brain barrier and lessening the side effects, such as nausea, caused by excess peripheral conversion of L-DOPA to dopamine.

There has been much debate about the wisdom of vitamin B6 supplementation in Parkinson's disease. This is due to concerns that peripheral dopamine levels may increase, lessening the amount of L-DOPA reaching the central nervous system, where it is needed for dopamine synthesis.

An alternative view is that carbidopa and benserazide may lead to an increase in neuronal issues, due to both these compounds being linked to a vitamin B6 deficiency. (Hinz et al. 2014).

In addition, carbidopa and benserazide may also be linked to a vitamin B3 deficiency, due to the inhibition of a B6-dependent enzyme in the kynurenine pathway. Blocking of the kynurenine pathway can lead to a significant drop in the synthesis of nicotinamide coenzymes (Bender et al. 1979). The kynurenine pathway is the metabolic pathway which the amino acid tryptophan takes to synthesise vitamin B3 in the body.

Plant sources of L-DOPA

A plant-source L-DOPA was first isolated from fava beans (broad beans) in 1913. In 1937 L-DOPA was discovered in the seeds of mucuna pruriens, a climbing legume found in India, Central and South America. Green beans and peas have also been found to contain L-DOPA.

Mucuna is thought to contain the highest natural source of L-DOPA, which acts in the plant as a natural insecticide. Interestingly, ayurvedic medicine has long described the use of mucuna or 'atmagupta' for nervous type maladies (Katzenschlager et al. 2004).

Fava beans have been reported to contain the aromatic amino acid decarboxylase inhibitor carbidopa, potentially increasing brain L-DOPA availability. To avoid flatulence, sprouted forms of the bean may be better tolerated (Mehran S M & B 2013).

Worryingly, excess fava bean ingestion has been linked to haemolytic anaemia (Leunbach et al. 2014). This dangerous side-effect of fava beans does effectively rule out their use for Parkinson's disease patients.

Misfolded Proteins – α-Synuclein

In Parkinson's, Alzheimer's, Huntingdon's, Motor Neurone and Creutzfeldt-Jakob diseases (CJD), misfolded proteins form a major part of the aetiology of each disease. Collectively, these diseases can all be considered to be *protein-misfolding diseases* (Drake 2015).

In a correctly folded protein, hydrophobic (repels water) amino acids are retained at the core of a protein. However, when a protein misfolds, hydrophobic amino acids are left exposed on the exterior of the protein and become vulnerable to adhering to other similar proteins, forming toxic aggregates and fibrils.

α-Synuclein and Parkinson's Disease

Unfolded or misfolded monomers of α-synuclein can form aggregates or oligomers when hydrophobic portions of the protein are exposed. Aggregates combine further, linking together to make sheets or fibrils. The fibrils then seed and induce the formation of Lewy bodies and Lewy neurites, leading to Parkinson's like pathology.

Lewy bodies and neurites are found in all Parkinson's disease brains and for this reason they are considered to be a signature pathology of the disease. A higher degree of Lewy bodies and neurites accumulating in Parkinson's disease brains, appears to correlate with a greater severity of symptoms and disability (Luk & Lee 2014).

The Braak hypothesis – are α-Synuclein aggregates able to seed?

Braak and colleagues in 2002 proposed 'The Braak hypothesis' where the early stages of the disease occur in areas outside of the substantia nigra and are largely asymptomatic. In stages 1 & 2, Lewy bodies and neurites are often seen in gastrointestinal, olfactory and cardiac neurons. It is not until stages 3 & 4 that the substantia nigra is affected and the classic motor symptoms appear.

Observations from the 'Braak hypothesis' suggest that Lewy body and neurite formation can occur in one part of the nervous system and slowly seed these aggregates to distant parts of the nervous system – and eventually to the substantia nigra (Luk & Lee 2014).

The Braak hypothesis is supported by findings that Parkinson's disease patients have been found not only to have increased intestinal α-synuclein, but additionally display increased intestinal permeability and mucosal staining for *E. coli* bacteria (Forsyth et al. 2011). This suggests that gastrointestinal inflammation and dysbiosis may lead to increased levels of misfolded α-synuclein within the enteric nervous system.

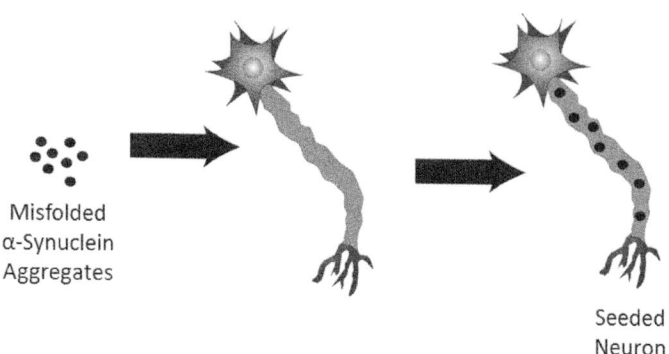

The 'seeding' of neurons with α-synuclein is the theory put forward by the Braak hypothesis

The Braak hypothesis puts forward the theory that it is the transmissibility of misfolded proteins which forms part of the aetiology of Parkinson's disease. This hypothesis is supported by the findings of transmission of prion proteins in Creutzfeldt-Jakob disease. Creutzfeldt-Jakob disease is a neurodegenerative condition triggered by the consumption of misfolded prion proteins from prion infected animal products.

Many animals are thought to become infected via prion-containing meat and bone meal products. Furthermore, nutrient-enhancing aluminosilicate additives in animal feeds may lead to increased transmission of prions within animals. Shockingly, these additives may increase prion transmission by as much as 680% (Johnson et al. 2011); (Kupfer et al. 2009).

Intact and modified α-Synuclein

Intact α-synuclein (in its soluble state) is thought to play an important role in dopamine storage vesicle activity, release of dopamine at synapses, calcium homeostasis and communication between the endoplasmic reticulum and mitochondria (Guardia-Laguarta et al. 2015).

On the other hand misfolded α-synuclein has been found to not only be insoluble, but to be post-translationally modified by phosphorylation, ubiquitination, nitrosylation and oxidation. When misfolded and modified, α-synuclein not only loses its function but also becomes toxic in its own right.

DOPAL, the toxic aldehyde produced during dopamine metabolism, can also lead to the formation of α-synuclein aggregates (Goldstein et al. 2013).

The post-translational modification of α-synuclein by phosphorylation is thought to lead to its increased aggregation and neurotoxicity. The enzyme protein phosphatase 2A (PP2A) can dephosphorylate α-synuclein and help protect against aggregation and fibril formation. Methylation of PP2A enhances its ability to dephosphorylate α-synuclein and decrease α-synuclein aggregation (Lee et al. 2013).

α-Synuclein degradation

α-Synuclein is normally degraded via the ubiquitin-proteasome system (UPS) and the autophagy-lysosome pathway (ALP). The activity of both these degradation pathways declines with age.

Although the processes are not totally understood, it is thought that the UPS manages increases in α-synuclein burden, and ALP clears pathogenic aggregates. The UPS may ubiquinate α-synuclein, but if unable to clear the protein, the ubiquitination may hinder subsequent ALP clearance (Xilouri et al. 2013).

Nutrition and α-Synuclein

Many plant polyphenols have been shown, in vivo, to be protective against α-synuclein fibrillation and aggregation. Some of the more effective compounds are:

Myricetin – from red wine, grapes, walnuts

EGCG (epigallocatechin gallate) – from green tea

Black tea extract – containing over 80% theaflavins

Curcumin – from turmeric

EGCG has the additional benefit of helping convert toxic α-synuclein fibrils into non-toxic aggregates (Caruana et al. 2011); (Ahmad & Lapidus 2012).

Eicosanoyl-5-hydroxytryptamide (EHT), a compound found in coffee, can help prevent PP2A demethylation thereby increasing its activity (Lee et al. 2011). Furthermore, coffee may exert protection in Parkinson's disease by two additional mechanisms. In the first, EHT may decrease microglial activation and associated neuroinflammation. In the second, caffeine inhibits adenosine A2A receptors, an action found to be protective for dopaminergic neurons (Lee et al. 2011). The caffeine content of 2 to 3 cups of coffee is thought to be safe but adverse effects such as anxiety, tremor, palpitation and potential bone loss, have to be considered (O'Keefe et al. 2013).

The binding of α-synuclein within lipid membranes is assisted by phospholipids with fatty acyl chains, such as DHA (Kubo et al. 2005). Caution must be exercised with polyunsaturated fatty acid supplementation since there is evidence that DHA may accelerate aggregate formation in the presence of α-synuclein (De Franceschi et al. 2011).

Lysosomal α-Synuclein Degradation

It is becoming clear that, to support correct α-synuclein function, every possible aspect of α-synuclein's metabolism will need to be fully explored. From synthesis, to degradation, its correct action and pathogenic action need to be addressed. Much of α-synuclein degradation should safely occur within an organelle called a lysosome.

Two important mechanisms for clearing α-synuclein are the ubiquitin proteasome system (UPS) and the autophagy-lysosome pathway (ALP) (Pan et al. 2008). The term autophagy literally means 'self-eating' (Yorimitsu & Klionsky 2005) and the idea that an organism can intentionally digest worn out cellular components has been gradually gaining acceptance amongst the scientific community. Failures of autophagy are now being found to be heavily implicated in neurodegenerative disease (Dall'Armi et al. 2013).

Autophagy and the Lysosome

There are three types of autophagy – macroautophagy, microautophagy and chaperone-mediated autophagy. Macroautophagy is considered the most important autophagic mechanism, and it is this subtype of autophagy that will be discussed.

The first step in the process of autophagy is when a lipid double-membrane wraps around a compound or organelle to form an autophagosome (Xilouri et al. 2013). In the next step, the autophagosome should ideally fuse with a type of organelle called a lysosome – but in Parkinson's disease this process often fails to occur or is dysfunctional.

One prominent feature of Parkinson's disease is the accumulation of autophagosomes, concomitant with lysosomal depletion, making it increasingly difficult to clear α-synuclein and other reactive proteins safely from dopaminergic neurons (Dehay et al. 2010).

Furthermore, it has been suggested that the export of α-synuclein into the extracellular space may occur when autophagy is dysfunctional, and that this could be one process which drives neurodegeneration (Takenouchi et al. 2009).

Lysosomal Breakdown

In an animal model, reactive oxygen species produced by defective mitochondria were found to breach lysosome membranes. This breach led to autophagosome accumulation, lysosomal breakdown and the release of lysosomal enzymes into the cytosol of neurons (Dehay et al. 2010).

ATP13A2 is an ATPase enzyme important in the correct function of lysosomes, and is therefore essential for the degradation of α-synuclein. Mutations in the *ATP13A2* gene (also known as *PARK9* gene) can lead to Kufor-Rakeb syndrome (KRS), a type of Parkinsonism.

Mutations or reduced function of ATP13A2 can lead to impaired clearance of lysosomal proteins, mitochondrial dysfunction, reduced lysosomal acidity (a low pH is required for lysosomal activity) and lowered autophagic flux (Holemans et al. 2015). Autophagic flux is a measure of the level of autophagy activation.

Heat Shock Protein 70.1, Calpain and Cathepsin

Hsp70.1 (heat shock protein 70.1) is a protein which protects lysosomal membranes, acts as a chaperone (by ensuring correct protein folding or digestion), and helps guard against cellular oxidative stress (Yamashima 2012); (Sahara & Yamashima 2010). Hsp70.1 is a substrate of the calcium-dependent protease, calpain.

Degradation of Hsp70.1 by calpain can lead to loss of lysosome integrity and the leakage of cathepsin proteases into the cytosol (Sahara & Yamashima 2010) in a process known as lysosome membrane permeabilisation (LMP). Cathepsin release from the lysosome into the cytosol can initiate cell death machinery and has led some observers to call lysosomes, 'suicide bags' (Appelqvist et al. 2013).

In another pathological mechanism, calpain has been shown to increase α-synuclein aggregation in animal models (Diepenbroek et al. 2014) and, in turn, α-synuclein aggregates have been suggested to lead to dysfunction of lysosomes (Chu et al. 2009).

Influx of calcium and dysregulation of calcium in a cell have the potential to activate calpain proteases excessively. Glutamate-mediated cellular excitotoxicity may, in part, be through calcium activation of calpain (Amadoro et al. 2006). The purine receptor P2X7 (once activated by extracellular ATP), can also trigger calcium-mediated calpain activity (Takenouchi et al. 2009); (Jiang et al. 2015).

Nutrition to Help Protect Lysosomes

The phospholipid phosphatidic acid (PA) is a product of the action of the enzyme phospholipase D2 on phosphatidylcholine (Dall'Armi et al. 2013). Phosphatidic acid can support the function of ATP13A2, and therefore could provide a protective role against α-synuclein toxicity and mitochondrial dysfunction in Parkinson's disease (Dall'Armi et al. 2013).

α-Synuclein had been found to suppress the activity of phospholipase D2 (Lotharius & Brundin 2002), suggesting that phosphatidic acid may be in short supply in Parkinson's disease brains. Frustratingly, α-synuclein has the ability to block its own degradation exactly at a time when lysosomes are needed to degrade toxic α-synuclein aggregates.

Vitamin B6, in its active form of pyridoxal 5'-phoshate (PLP), has been shown to display neuroprotective properties in primates by inhibiting the activity of cathepsins. PLP was found to bind to and inhibit the cysteine residues of cathepsins released from lysosomes, due to calpain-induced dysfunction (Yamashima et al. 2001).

Mitochondria and Parkinson's Disease

What are mitochondria?

Mitochondria are multi-functional organelles, well-known for their vital role in energy production. Mitochondria also play an important role in cellular calcium balance, cell fate decisions, oxygen sensing, hormone synthesis, haeme synthesis, and form part of the immune system's defence against pathogens (Nunnari & Suomalainen 2012); (Bell et al. 2007); (Strushkevich et al. 2011).

Mitochondria and evolution

Mitochondria first appeared around 1.8 billion years ago when aerobic and anaerobic organisms symbiotically combined to produce eukaryotic cells or eukaryotes. Eukaryotes are the cellular building blocks of all complex life forms (Martin & Mentel 2010).

How do mitochondria produce ATP?

To produce aerobic energy, mitochondria extract energy from food via the tricarboxylic cycle and the electron transport chain (ETC). The ETC is a mechanism within mitochondria which transfers high energy electrons from NADH (produced in the tricarboxylic acid cycle), to pump hydrogen ions into the intermembrane space. It is the re-entry of hydrogen ions, through complex V of the ETC, which transfers energy from ADP (adenosine diphosphate) to ATP (adenosine triphosphate). ATP is the main energy currency of a cell (Nunnari & Suomalainen 2012).

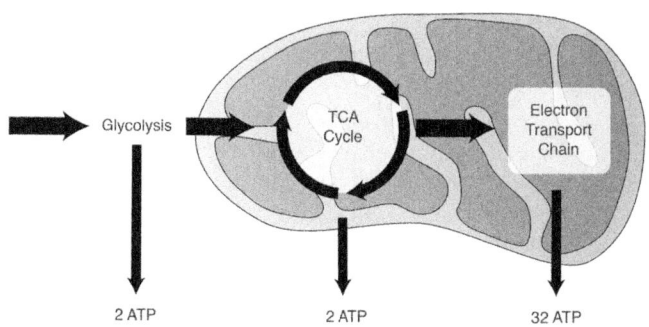

Mitochondria can produce 34 molecules of ATP from a single molecule of glucose.

Mitochondria travel on tracks along the axon of a neuron

Mitochondria are dynamic and motile (mobile) organelles which are constantly fusing and dividing to help maintain mitochondrial integrity. Within a cell, mitochondria travel on cytoskeletal tracks, driven by protein motors, to reach areas of energetic need. Cytoskeletal tracks are of particular importance for neurons because of the comparatively long distances between nucleus and synapse in many of these cells (Perier & Vila 2012).

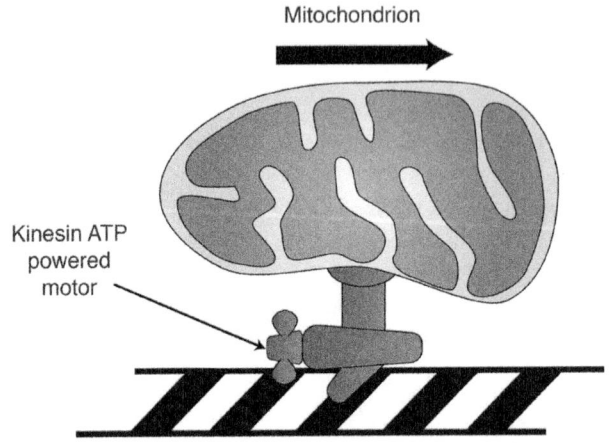

A mitochondrion travels along a cytoskeletal track within the axon of a neuron, powered by a kinesin protein ATP-powered motor.

How are mitochondria implicated in Parkinson's disease?

Neurons are extremely vulnerable to impaired function when synaptic mitochondrial complex I activity of the ETC falls below approximately 25% of normal (Mattson & Liu 2002). Away from the synapse, brain complex I activity can fall by around 70% before damaging effects occur (Berman & Hastings 2001).

Many researchers (and Parkinson's disease patients themselves) are acutely aware that low energy levels exacerbate their symptoms, and that a general level of fatigue may accompany the disease (Lou et al. 2001).

Improving mitochondrial function and ATP synthesis can be a double-edged sword for Parkinson's disease patients, since injured mitochondria are programmed to initiate a cell death process called apoptosis; in Parkinson's disease some degree of anaerobic respiration may therefore be protective (Johansen et al. 2010).

Mitochondria are thought to be capable of producing large quantities of ROS and RNS (Turrens 2003), and so that optimising their function may lessen the chances of neuronal damage and help increase energy production.

There are five complexes in the ETC but, as mentioned above, it is complex I at the very start of the ETC that is often blocked or dysfunctional in Parkinson's disease (Keeney et al. 2006). With complex I blocked, high energy electrons may leave the ETC and combine with oxygen to form the damaging radical, superoxide (Turrens 2003).

Compounds known to block complex I are the protein aggregates of α-synuclein, the pesticide rotenone, nitric oxide, peroxynitrite and quinone metabolites of dopamine (Devi et al. 2008); (Tanner et al. 2011); (Chinta & Andersen 2011); (Ben-Shachar et al. 2002).

Nutrition and mitochondria

There are many nutrients which can both support mitochondrial function and help protect mitochondria against dysfunction. Magnesium, lipoic acid and the whole gamut of B vitamins are required to maintain the activity of the tricarboxylic acid cycle. The electron transport chain requires, B2, B3, magnesium, iron, sulphur, glutathione, cysteine and CoQ10 (Pieczenik & Neustadt 2007).

Astaxanthin and ascorbate can help protect mitochondria from oxidative stress (Wolf et al. 2010); (Li et al. 2001) and taurine has been found to regulate mitochondrial protein synthesis in addition to its antioxidant activity (Jong et al. 2012).

Resveratrol and quercetin can help stimulate the biogenesis of new mitochondria (Sun et al. 2010); (Davis et al. 2009).

Compounds in broccoli and turmeric can help protect mitochondria by up-regulating the synthesis of antioxidant enzymes. These plant compounds up-regulate enzymes such as glutathione S-transferase, via the activation of the transcription factor Nrf2 and the nuclear antioxidant response element (ARE) (Innamorato et al. 2008); (Wu et al. 2013).

The antioxidant hormone melatonin helps to maintain mitochondrial function. Melatonin is preferentially taken up by mitochondria and so underlines the importance of adequate sleep to help preserve mitochondrial function (Srinivasan et al. 2011).

Losses in ATP production can lead to neuronal death. It is thought that highly toxic misfolded prion proteins exert their effects through depletion of nicotinamide adenine dinucleotide (NAD^+) resulting in an energy crisis (Zhou et al. 2015). It therefore seems likely that replenishment with supplemental NAD^+ may also help protect against dopaminergic neuron death when exposed to α-synuclein.

α-Synuclein and Fatigue

α-Synuclein is thought to be up-regulated when cells are exposed to low levels of toxicity and oxidative stress, possibly as a protective measure against apoptosis. Pathogenic accumulation of α-synuclein into aggregates and Lewy bodies is thought to be secondary to the initial protective action of the protein (Musgrove et al. 2011).

Is α-synuclein responsible for cancer-related fatigue?

In a study observing radiation-related fatigue in cancer patients, it was found that radiation exposure induced increased expression of α-synuclein, concomitant with the appearance of fatigue symptoms. Moreover, neurological dysfunction is a common symptom in cancer patients and α-synuclein may play a role (Saligan et al. 2013).

It is highly likely therefore, that radiation-induced oxidative stress may lead to increased expression of α-synuclein, initially as a protective measure. The study findings do allude to how oxidative stress in Parkinson's disease patients could lead to pathological expression of α-synuclein and Parkinson's disease-related fatigue.

α-Synuclein and mitochondrial dysfunction

α-Synuclein is able to be imported into mitochondria via voltage-dependent anion channels (VDACs). Once inside the outer mitochondrial membrane, α-synuclein is then able to block the activity of VDACs, leading to a reduction in vital metabolites passing in and out of a mitochondrion (Rostovtseva et al. 2015).

In animal models of Parkinson's disease, α-synuclein over-expression causes the down-regulation of both complex I and complex IV of the mitochondrial electron transport chain (Zhang et al. 2013).

In Alzheimer's disease, amyloid-β proteins can bind to and inhibit mitochondrial complex IV by attaching to the haeme moiety of the complex. Like amyloid-β, α-synuclein has an affinity for haeme, suggesting that it may inhibit complex IV in a similar manner. Furthermore, haeme has been shown to protect against the aggregation of α-synuclein, and potentially even reverse the process (Hayden et al. 2015).

Haeme deficiency and neurodegeneration

Haeme deficiency increases with ageing and in neurodegenerative disease. It is associated with reduced mitochondrial complex IV activity, increased nitric oxide synthase expression and dysregulated iron and zinc metabolism. Vitamin B6, iron, lipoic acid and zinc are all required for haeme synthesis (Atamna et al. 2002). Conversely, manganese, mercury, lead, cadmium, (Medlock et al. 2009) aluminium (Atamna et al. 2002) and salicylic acid (Gupta et al. 2013) can block its synthesis through disruption of the enzyme ferrochelatase. Ferrochelatase is a mitochondrial enzyme which inserts iron into a protoporphyrin structure as the final step in haeme synthesis.

Frustratingly, the addition of dietary red meat and haeme may be counterproductive in Parkinson's disease, due to the overexpression of the enzyme haeme oxygenase-1 (HO-1). HO-1 degrades haeme to free iron which is also implicated in Parkinson's disease pathology (Schipper et al. 2009).

In Alzheimer's disease, an amyloid-β –haeme complex acts as an agent of peroxidation, potentially increasing oxidative stress (Atamna 2006); it is possible, therefore, that α-synuclein-haeme complexes could also increase oxidative stress. An interesting area of future research would be to see whether other haeme-like porphyrin structures, such as vitamin B12 and chlorophyll, could help protect α-synuclein from aggregation.

Salicylic acid inhibition of ferrochelatase does raise some concerns about excessive use of Aspirin (acetylsalicylic acid) in Parkinson's disease. On the one hand, Aspirin may reduce neuroinflammation but, worryingly, it could undermine mitochondrial function and ATP synthesis.

The Endoplasmic Reticulum

What is the endoplasmic reticulum?

The endoplasmic reticulum (ER) is a labyrinthine network of membranes forming a cellular organelle which acts as a 'processing plant' for many proteins and lipids.

The ER and mitochondria work together to maintain cellular calcium homeostasis; calcium concentrations within the ER are estimated to be 100-fold higher than within the cytosol (Marcoux et al. 2002).

The ER is involved in protein synthesis, folding, post-translational modification and transport (Lindholm et al. 2006).

The ER, alongside the Golgi apparatus, is a major site for both lipid and phospholipid synthesis (Fagone & Jackowski 2009). Feedback control of cholesterol synthesis is dependent on the ER.

HMG CoA reductase, the rate-limiting enzyme for cholesterol synthesis, is sited in ER membranes. When sterols accumulate in ER membranes, a process is triggered to degrade HMG CoA reductase, neatly providing negative feedback for control of cholesterol synthesis (Jo & Debose-Boyd 2010).

How is the ER implicated in Parkinson's disease?

There are an increasing number of papers supporting the ER's role in Parkinson's disease, leading some researchers to suggest adopting an *"ERcentric view of Parkinson's disease"* (Mercado et al. 2013).

Much of the recent research on Parkinson's disease has focussed on the role that dysfunctional mitochondria play in the aetiology of the disease. The endoplasmic reticulum (ER) is an organelle that is less well-known than the mitochondrion, but is equally important when considering cellular dysfunction in Parkinson's disease.

These two organelles work in very close association, particularly when working to buffer calcium actions within the cell. Excess calcium release into the cytosol can be problematic in a neuron, leading to many damaging reactions. The storage of calcium in the ER and mitochondrion can buffer or protect a neuron from these damaging reactions (Surmeier et al. 2011).

The ER and mitochondria are bound via the mitochondria-associated ER membrane (MAM) (Guardia-Laguarta et al. 2014). α-Synuclein is a component of the MAM and plays an integral role in calcium transfer between the two organelles. Increased expression of α-synuclein, or increased aggregation, may lead to disruption of this calcium transfer and consequent loss of mitochondrial function (Calì et al. 2012).

Inflammation, infection, increases in α-synuclein expression and other triggers, can lead to ER stress and activation of the ER unfolded protein response (UPR) (Drake 2015). The UPR is a mechanism which normally triggers the removal or repair of misfolded proteins. Increased expression of α-synuclein may overwhelm the ER UPR, leading to neuronal apoptosis (Bernales et al. 2012).

Nutrition and the ER

As a major site of protein and lipid synthesis, the ER requires adequate dietary amino acids and fatty acid intake. Protein folding within the ER is dependent on the oxidation of protein in a tightly-controlled redox environment. Glutathione, ascorbate, riboflavin, vitamin K and tocopherol all assist in the process of protein folding.

Studies have shown that ascorbate deficiency can result in ER stress and activation of the unfolded protein response, suggesting that some of the symptoms of scurvy may be due to ER stress (Margittai et al. 2005); (Bánhegyi et al. 2003) (Rutkevich & Williams 2012). Lion's Mane mushroom has been found to protect against ER stress, promote neurite outgrowth and help prevent neuronal apoptosis (Lai et al. 2013).

The Benzene Ring, Health and Disease

Living systems have to be able to harness the positive aspects of unstable minerals and compounds to allow for a multitude of life-giving biochemical processes. Keeping instability within limits is important for health, but, when out of control, many degenerative diseases such as Parkinson's disease can occur.

One volatile organic compound is benzene, which is formed from a ring of carbon atoms and called a benzene ring. Benzene is a highly toxic component of many petrochemicals. A benzene ring within a compound gives it the label of an aromatic hydrocarbon as many compounds containing a benzene ring have a strong aroma. Not all compounds with a benzene ring are toxic, and plant polyphenols and the amino acids phenylalanine and tyrosine contain them.

The chemical symbol for the benzene ring

If benzene is hydroxylated (as in the above configuration) it becomes known as a catechol

The neurotransmitter dopamine is a catecholamine because of the catechol within its structure

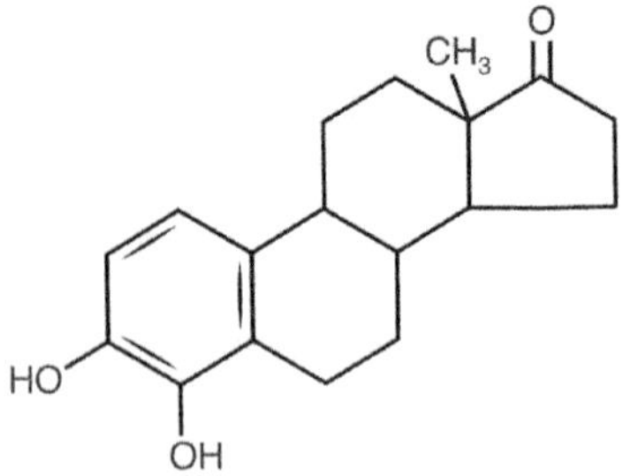

4-hydroxyestrone is a catechol oestrogen which forms genotoxic DNA adducts. Note the hydroxylated benzene ring which it has in common with dopamine

Volatile organic compounds may deplete antioxidants

From the above diagrams we can see that the benzene ring is at the heart of dopamine, oestrogens and catechol oestrogens. Hopefully, it is now even more apparent how toxic volatile organic compounds can compromise the metabolism of these important endogenous hydrocarbons. It is the similar structure of toxic and endogenous compounds which allows the toxic compounds to undermine and interfere with endogenous compounds and their receptors.

Toxic volatile organic compounds are thought to deplete cellular antioxidants, leaving a person unable to metabolise normal oestrogen and dopamine hydrocarbon metabolites from the endocrine and nervous systems.

Plant polyphenols and Parkinson's disease

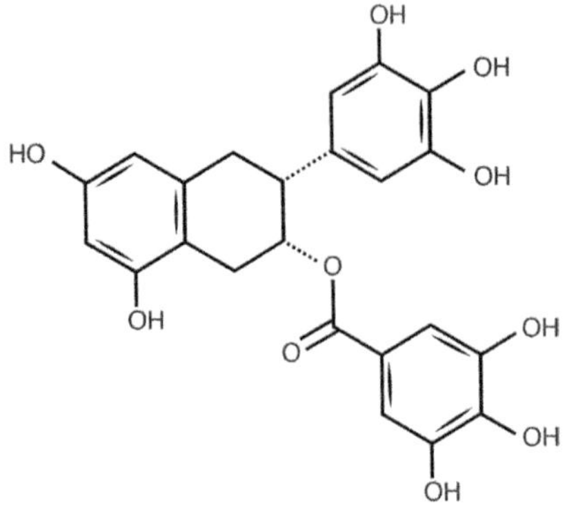

Green and black tea contain polyphenols called catechins. The most well-studied and abundant catechin in tea is epigallocatechin gallate (EGCG), depicted at the foot of the previous page. Note the catechol component on the far left of the diagram. It is interesting how protective green tea is in Parkinson's disease, particularly since both dopamine and green tea contain catechols.

Curcumin and resveratrol are further examples of polyphenols, both found to be protective against Parkinson's disease.

The aryl hydrocarbon receptor and aromatic compounds

Exogenous and endogenous aromatic compounds are ligands of the aryl hydrocarbon receptor. The aryl hydrocarbon receptor is responsible for the expression of CYP1B1, the enzyme which transforms oestrogen to its genotoxic 4-hydroxyestrone metabolite.

The aryl hydrocarbon receptor also has an influence on tyrosine hydroxylase, the rate-limiting enzyme for dopamine synthesis. Activation of the aryl hydrocarbon receptor by the environmental toxin dioxin, has been found to alter the expression of tyrosine hydroxylase (Akahoshi et al. 2009). Moreover, microglia within the CNS contain aryl hydrocarbon receptors which modify the microglial response to bacterial endotoxins (Lee et al. 2015).

Resveratrol has been shown to be an inhibitor of the aryl hydrocarbon receptor and curcumin and quercetin may weakly bind the aryl hydrocarbon receptor. These natural polyphenols all act to limit over-activation of the aryl hydrocarbon receptor by xenobiotic aromatic compounds (Xiao 2015).

In summary, this chapter highlights the essential role that plant polyphenols can play in helping balance endogenous aromatic compounds against the damaging impact of xenobiotic aromatic compounds. It is the similarity in chemical structure between polyphenols and dopamine and oestrogen metabolites which can provide this protection.

Fatty Acids – A new understanding

A paradigm shift in the science of fatty acids

For many years, fats and fatty acids have been viewed simply as dietary compounds which supply calories for energy production. Many people obsessively avoid dietary fat in fear of potential weight gain. This outdated view is now proving to be woefully inadequate since more and more studies are starting to reveal the complexity of these highly metabolically-active compounds.

In addition to being an energy source, fatty acids can help build cell membranes, control gene expression, trigger and resolve inflammation, and modify protein behaviour and activity. Protein modification by fatty acids is also known as post-translational modification, since fatty acids can alter protein behaviour after protein synthesis (many other compounds can do this, including ROS and nitric oxide).

Not all fats are born equal

Saturated fat is a generic term that fails to describe the variety of behaviours displayed by different chain lengths of saturated fatty acids. When working with a highly complex condition such Parkinson's disease, it is essential to be able to differentiate between different types of saturated fatty acids. Examples of saturated fatty acids are butyrate, caprylate, laurate, myristate and palmitate; all having completely different behaviours and functions.

Polyunsaturated and monounsaturated fatty acids (PUFAs and MUFAs) have their own multitude of configurations with diverse metabolic effects within the CNS (central nervous system). An example of this paradigm-shift in understanding of fats and fatty acids is the perception of the lipid droplet. The lipid droplet was initially perceived as a passive intracellular lipid store, but, over time, it has now come to be recognised as a highly dynamic organelle, pro-actively functioning to help manage intracellular and membrane lipids (Beller et al. 2010).

Neuroprotective aspects of PUFAs

A diet high in polyunsaturated fatty acids has been suggested to be protective against Parkinson's disease (de Lau et al. 2005).

The most promising polyunsaturated fatty acid in relation to Parkinson's disease is the omega-3 fatty acid, docosahexaenoic acid (DHA). DHA is essential for the development of the brain, is anti-inflammatory, increases glutathione synthesis, reduces apoptosis in dopaminergic neurons and helps decrease L-DOPA-related dyskinesia in laboratory animals (Seidl et al. 2014).

Omega-3 fatty acids are required for the synthesis of a family of compounds known as *'Pro-resolving lipid mediators'*. The mediators include resolvin, protectin, neuroprotectin and maresin. The resolution of inflammation, infection and the enabling of tissue repair, are reported to be amongst their many functions (Serhan 2014).

One neuroprotective lipid mediator is the DHA-dependent nervous system sentinel, neuroprotectin D1 (NPD1). NPD1 synthesis is induced in response to protein misfolding and helps to protect neurons from apoptosis. NPD1 may also work as a modulator of the enzyme protein phosphatase 2A (PP2A), the enzyme linked with dephosphorylating α-synuclein and reducing aggregate formation (Bazan 2013).

Resolvin D1 (RvD1) is a DHA-dependent anti-inflammatory lipid mediator. RvD1 is able to suppress inflammatory cytokine expression in microglia, thus providing protection from neuroinflammation (Xu et al. 2013).

DHA and EPA are natural agonists for the nuclear receptor PPAR-γ (peroxisome proliferator-activated receptor gamma) (Grygiel-Górniak 2014). PPAR-γ in turn may act as a regulator of microglial-associated neuroinflammation (Bernardo & Minghetti 2006). Another novel role for PPAR-γ is as a regulator of the expression of the insulin-degrading enzyme (IDE), an enzyme which forms protective complexes with α-synuclein (Du et al. 2009).

There has been much debate about the most effective way of increasing DHA levels in humans. Dietary and supplementary α-linolenic acid (ALA) and EPA can increase blood levels of EPA, but these fatty acids are thought to have very little effect on blood DHA levels (Brenna et al. 2009). In most people there is poor enzymatic conversion from ALA to DHA, frequently with only 3-4% of ALA being metabolised to DHA. A diet rich in omega-6 PUFAs can reduce this conversion by a further 40-50% (Gerster 1998). Supplementary DHA may be the only way to significantly increase blood DHA status (Brenna et al. 2009). Additionally, there is some evidence that the plant polyphenol curcumin may accelerate the synthesis of DHA from its precursor ALA (α-linolenic acid) (Wu et al. 2015).

The effect of DHA on monoamine oxidase activity

Age-related increases in the activity of the enzyme monoamine oxidase can decrease brain dopamine and increase DOPAL, dopamine's toxic metabolite. In animal models, DOPAL has been found to lower dietary and brain levels of omega-3 fatty acids (particularly DHA). This can lead to increases in MAO-B activity, with concomitant decreases in dopamine in some brain regions. In another study, DHA has been reported to decrease MAO activity by around 40%, with a high-fat diet accelerating MAO activity by approximately 25% (Di Lisa et al. 2014).

The enzyme MAO is attached to the fatty outer mitochondrial membrane. Could DHA help maintain dopamine levels by interfering with MAO's attachment?

The integrity of vesicle membranes is important for safe cellular storage of dopamine. Omega-3 fatty acids may help support vesicle membranes since omega-3 deficiency has been found to reduce VMAT2 activity, leading to depletion of dopamine in storage vesicles (Müller et al. 2014).

Many of the above studies are cell-based or animal-based studies. If they can translate to Parkinson's disease patients then omega-3 fatty acids could help to decrease toxic DOPAL and increase the safe storage of dopamine in vesicles.

DHA can increase the threshold of immune system activation

Toll-like receptors (TLRs) are pattern recognition receptors of the innate immune system which recognise fragments of bacteria, such as lipopolysaccharide (LPS). LPS can act as an agonist for TLR4, leading to activation of microglia within the CNS. Microglia, under LPS stimulation, produce neurotoxic inflammatory cytokines and the excitotoxin glutamate (Trudler et al. 2010).

DHA can inhibit TLR4 recruitment into lipid rafts, suggesting another anti-inflammatory mechanism for this PUFA (Wong et al. 2009). Outside of the CNS, PUFAs can modify the SFA content of lipid rafts in T cells, to exert an immunosuppressive, anti-inflammatory effect (Stulnig 1998).

Unlike DHA, the saturated fatty acid laurate has been reported to increase the sensitivity of TLR4 to LPS by recruiting TLR4 into lipid rafts and activating downstream inflammatory pathways. Laurate is the main fatty acid in coconut oil and so may be more inflammatory than many people realise.

Negative aspects of PUFAs

Polyunsaturated fats (PUFAs), such as DHA and EPA, are extremely vulnerable to lipid peroxidation and, in excess, could render neurons vulnerable to apoptosis (Liu et al. 2008). Worryingly, there is some evidence that DHA may accelerate aggregate formation in the presence of α-synuclein (De Franceschi et al. 2011).

Alternatively, other research has found that an increase in red blood cell DHA concentration can help reduce lipid peroxidation markers (Shichiri et al. 2014). The body can normally protect against oxidised lipids by inducing Nrf2 (nuclear factor E2-relatedfactor 2), a transcription factor that helps to up-regulate endogenous antioxidant synthesis, when exposed to oxidising compounds (Gruber et al. 2015).

It might be wise therefore, to supplement plant phenolic compounds such as curcumin alongside PUFAs. Curcumin has been found not only to induce Nrf2, but also to reduce defective signalling of Nrf2, which may improve endogenous antioxidant synthesis (He et al. 2012).

Research on omega-6 PUFAs and Parkinson's disease is contradictory, possibly because the many different sub-types and effects of fatty acids are not completely defined. The main omega-6 PUFA in the brain is arachidonic acid (AA).

In Parkinson's disease subjects, brain lipid raft AA is reduced by 60% and DHA by 75% (Fabelo et al. 2011), but dietary addition of AA is likely to be unwise (Miyake et al. 2010). This is because AA, released from phospholipids by the enzyme phospholipase A2 (PLA2), can take part in the AA cascade, where AA acts as a substrate for inflammatory cyclooxygenase enzymes (COX-1 and COX-2).

Increased COX enzyme activity has been linked to altered dopaminergic signalling, microglial activation and neurodegeneration (Lee et al. 2010); (Teismann 2012). EPA, the omega-3 PUFA and vitamin E can both act as an inhibitors of PLA2 and so help protect against PUFA loss from lipid rafts (Song et al. 2006); (Farooqui 2006). Curcumin and sesamin from turmeric, and sesame oil can both inhibit the delta 5-desaturaturation of omega-6 fatty acids, blocking AA synthesis (Fujiyama-Fujiwara et al. 1992).

Aside from the omega-6 fatty acid association with the AA cascade, excessive dietary omega-6 intake may lead to displacement of omega-3 fatty acids from lipid rafts (Ma et al. 2004). As mentioned above, another important benefit of curcumin synergy with PUFAs is that it has been shown to accelerate the synthesis of DHA from its precursor ALA (α-linolenic acid) (Wu et al. 2015).

Phosphatidylserine – good or bad?

Phosphatidylserine (PS) is an intracellular phospholipid that forms a vital part in the mechanism of binding α-synuclein into lipid rafts. To be effective, PS requires either DHA or AA as fatty acyl chains within the phospholipid (Kubo et al. 2015).

Furthermore, DHA has been reported to enhance phosphatidylserine synthesis (Bazinet & Layé 2014).

In a similar way to AA, displaced PS may trigger destructive processes. PS outside a cell acts as an "eat-me" signal to enable phagocytosis of a neuron by microglia (Neher et al. 2013). It might be unwise to supplement PS in neurodegenerative disease if there is a risk of supplemental PS activating microglia. Many PS supplements are of soy phospholipid origin and will not have DHA as a fatty acyl chain. The FDA in America states:

"Bovine brain cortex and soy-based phosphatidyl serine are different substances and might, therefore, have different biological activities. Thus, there is considerable uncertainty in generalising results from studies done with bovine brain cortex phosphatidyl serine as the test substance to soy-based phosphatidyl serine, and vice versa (FDA, 2003)."

Saturated fats, palmitate and protein modification

Saturated fatty acids such as palmitate, laurate, and stearate can increase CNS inflammatory cytokine synthesis (Hussain et al. 2013), with palmitate and stearate being found to be increased in Parkinson's disease brains (Kubo et al. 2015).

In addition, palmitate may disrupt blood-brain barrier function (Takechi et al. 2013). Avoidance of dietary palmitate may not protect the CNS as de novo synthesis can provide substantial amounts of palmitate through the enzyme fatty acid synthase (FASN).

A low-fat, high-carbohydrate diet may lead to increases in de novo palmitate synthesis, since the body is designed to store high glucose intakes as fat, via activation of FASN.

Insulin resistance, obesity and type 2 diabetes are all linked to over-expression of FASN known as a 'lipogenic state' (Menendez et al. 2009). In animals fed an omega-3 PUFA-rich diet, gene expression of FASN was found to be suppressed (Teran-Garcia et al. 2007).

Protein palmitoylation, or protein S-acylation, is a form of lipidation that reversibly modifies cysteine residues of proteins to help target them to lipid domains. Palmitate modification permits the tethering of a protein in the cholesterol and sphingomyelin-rich lipid domain and increases protein activity (Wan et al. 2007).

BAX (Bcl-2-associated X protein) is a cytosolic proapoptotic protein linked to dopaminergic neuron death. To initiate apoptosis, BAX associates with mitochondrial outer membranes, a process that requires palmitate modification to BAX via palmitoylation.

Decreasing BAX palmitoylation can reduce the translocation of BAX from the cytosol to mitochondria, and could help protect dopaminergic neurons (Fröhlich et al. 2014); (Charan et al. 2014).

Inducible nitric oxide synthase (iNOS) is a nitric oxide-producing enzyme found to be highly expressed in the substantia nigra of Parkinson's disease cases (Kavyaa & Dikshit 2005). In a similar way to BAX, iNOS requires palmitoylation before it can be targeted to intracellular domains.

Endothelial nitric oxide synthase (eNOS) requires similar modifications to enable the enzyme to help maintain healthy blood pressure, highlighting the importance of palmitoylation. Problems only occur when palmitoylation modifies an excess number of proteins (Kim & Ross 2014).

Ketogenic diets have been reported to provide symptomatic relief for almost half of Parkinson's disease patients consuming high fat foods for 28 days (Gasior et al. 2006). It may be wise for Parkinson's patients to be cautious about the long-chain saturated fat content of a ketogenic diet, due to the negative effects of SFAs, such as palmitate.

Olive oil and neuroprotection

Olive oil is a rich source of MUFAs and has been found to play a protective role in Parkinson's disease. Animal sources of MUFA have not been found to be as beneficial as olive oil MUFAs (Schwingshackl & Hoffmann 2014) suggesting that the polyphenol component provides many of olive oil's protective qualities. Extra virgin olive oil is rich in the polyphenols oleuropein and hydroxytyrosol, both found to decrease oxidative damage in the substantia nigra of laboratory animals (Sarbishegi et al. 2014).

Cholesterol and Parkinson's Disease – Contradictory Evidence

Many studies have found both positive and negative associations between cholesterol metabolism and Parkinson's disease, but the complexity of the relationship has been extremely difficult to unravel. A major stumbling block had been the demonisation of cholesterol by the medical world. In the race to lower cholesterol levels, the subtleties of CNS (central nervous system) cholesterol metabolism, and the brain's need for significant amounts of lipids to maintain neuronal integrity, may have been lost.

Furthermore, Parkinson's disease is an age-related condition and low cholesterol in the elderly has been associated with increases in all-cause mortality (Schatz et al. 2001). HMG-CoA reductase (the rate-limiting enzyme for synthesis of cholesterol and target of statin drugs) resides in the ER (endoplasmic reticulum) membrane (Burg & Espenshade 2011). Stresses within the ER may, therefore, have a negative impact on cholesterol metabolism.

Cholesterol Metabolism and Parkinson's disease

Paradoxically, some studies find an association between high dietary cholesterol and saturated fat and Parkinson's disease, and others find no association with serum cholesterol levels (Rantham Prabhakara et al. 2008). The age of the study cohorts may be a factor in the conflicting results of studies, or it could be that cholesterol-lowering strategies are only preventative against Parkinson's disease in adults younger than 60 years of age.

Moreover, the protective effects of cholesterol lowering may be due to the secondary effects of statins, such as reductions in oxidative stress, α-synuclein and inflammatory cytokine expression, and not due to cholesterol reduction per se (Gao 2012). Confusing the issue even further, some statins are more lipophilic than others; that is, they may more easily cross into the brain and have stronger cholesterol-lowering effects in the CNS than hydrophilic statin drugs.

The brain contains about a quarter of total body cholesterol, and due to the blood-brain barrier (BBB) much of this cholesterol is synthesised locally, making the brain largely independent of liver-derived cholesterol (Björkhem et al. 2013). Cholesterol cannot cross the BBB, but oxidised cholesterol in the form of oxysterol can cross the barrier.

The main CNS oxysterol is 24S-hydroxycholesterol, found to be protective for the activity of tyrosine hydroxylase, the rate-limiting enzyme for dopamine synthesis (Rantham Prabhakara et al. 2008). When the BBB is compromised, excessive peripheral 27-hydroxycholesterol may cross the BBB.

27-hydroxycholesterol is an oxysterol that has been associated with increased α-synuclein, neuronal apoptosis and decreased tyrosine hydroxylase expression.

Increased 27-hydroxycholesterol has been found in the brains of Parkinson's disease patients and, along with other oxysterols, is associated with Multiple Sclerosis, Huntingdon's disease and Alzheimer's disease. 27-hydroxycholesterol is thought to act an oestrogen receptor antagonist, thereby blocking oestrogen receptor beta (ERβ)-induced tyrosine hydroxylase expression (Marwarha et al. 2011).

The mitochondria-associated ER membrane (MAM) contains cholesterol-rich lipid rafts. α-Synuclein has a high affinity for lipid rafts, probably due to its two cholesterol-binding domains. It is thought that disruption to cholesterol and α-synuclein metabolism within the MAM may be an early event in the pathology that leads to Parkinson's disease. Researchers are calling this line of thought the "MAM hypothesis" (Guardia-Laguarta et al. 2015).

Nutrition, Cholesterol and Parkinson's Disease

High consumption of β-Sitosterol, a plant sterol rich in nuts, seeds, vegetable oils and avocado, has been shown to lead to the degeneration of dopaminergic neurons in laboratory animals. It is thought that β-Sitosterol may excessively activate cholesterol efflux from neurons, leading to cholesterol depletion, and dopaminergic neuronal degeneration (Kim et al. 2008). It is unlikely that general consumption of sterol-rich foods would undermine neuronal function, but sterol supplementation could be potentially problematic.

Coenzyme Q10 is a mitochondrial coenzyme which is dependent on cholesterol metabolism. Statins may decrease the synthesis of coenzyme Q10 and could, therefore, undermine mitochondrial function (Marcoff & Thompson 2007).

Many phytoestrogens act as agonists for ERβ, the oestrogen receptor shown to promote neuronal survival. In animal models, the soy-derived phytoestrogens genistein, daidzein and equol have proven to display neuroprotective properties, without displaying feminising activity (Zhao et al. 2013).

Lipid Rafts

Many proteins and enzymes require a rigid platform within a membrane for them to function appropriately. Normal lipid membranes can be too fluid to provide this platform but lipid rafts, enriched with cholesterol and sphingolipids, can provide an ideal platform for proteins and enzymes. α-Synuclein function is very closely associated with lipid rafts, so to fully understand α-synuclein, it is important to pay close attention to these fatty microdomains.

Lipid rafts may be seen as firm microdomains floating within fluid membranes (Staubach & Hanisch 2011). Modification of proteins by a saturated fat such as palmitate, can assist the targeting and tethering of proteins to a lipid raft. Once tethered with palmitate, the activity of a protein may increase (Bhattacharyya et al. 2013).

Modification of membranes by dietary lipids is emerging as an area of increasing interest, since, in Parkinson's disease, many proteins or enzymes associated with the aetiology of the disease, are found to be tethered to lipid rafts.

Furthermore, interaction of some of the main protagonists in Parkinson's disease, occur in lipid rafts. The endoplasmic reticulum, α-synuclein, and mitochondria all have vital roles associated with these fatty microdomains.

Lipid rafts are essential for immune system communication

Lipid rafts act as important signalling domains not just for the nervous system but also for the function of T-cells, B-cells (Simons & Toomre 2000), cytokines (Li et al. 2005), immunoglobulins (Weise et al. 2011), macrophages (George & Wu 2012) and receptors for glycated proteins (Wang et al. 2015).

The altered activity of lipid rafts is associated with the up-regulation of immunoglobulin IgE and may predispose an individual to increased sensitivity to allergy. Age-related changes in lipid raft fatty acid content may make microglia in the brain more reactive to glycated proteins (AGEs). Increasingly, the anti-inflammatory omega-3 polyunsaturated fatty acid (PUFA) DHA (docosahexaenoic acid) is being found positively to modulate all the above immune-related components and their receptors.

Lipid rafts are also found in microglia (the resident macrophages of the CNS) (Faustino et al. 2011), foam cells in blood vessels (Schmitz & Grandl 2007) and osteoclasts in bone (Ryu et al. 2010). Lipid rafts may therefore reveal some answers relating to neurodegenerative disease, atherosclerosis and osteoporosis.

Lipid rafts and Parkinson's disease

There is a close connection between lipid rafts and many proteins and complexes associated with Parkinson's disease. These include α-synuclein, LRRK2 (Leucine-rich repeat kinase 2), Parkin, DJ-1 (Kubo et al. 2015), the MAM and dopaminergic microglia (Hicks et al. 2012). The close association of lipid rafts with these complexes and proteins makes them of particular interest in Parkinson's disease - possibly indicating that lipid raft disturbances may be another signature of the disease.

Modification of lipid rafts – negative effects of palmitate

Many lipid raft proteins are post-translationally modified by the binding of palmitate, known as palmitoylation.

It may be that DHA and other PUFAs could positively modify lipid raft activity by antagonising palmitoylation (Ma et al. 2004).

In the pancreatic beta cell, palmitate excess leads to lipotoxicity through palmitate antagonising lipid raft sphingomyelin and initiating ER stress (Boslem et al. 2013). If this mechanism translates to dopaminergic neurons, it would be wise to avoid dietary long-chain SFAs in Parkinson's disease.

Lipid rafts have been found to play a role in Alzheimer's disease. In experiments, palmitoylation of the amyloid precursor protein (APP) led to a doubling of amyloid-β production; palmitoylation of APP leads to an increased affinity of the protein to lipid rafts, where the protein can be cleaved to form amyloid-β (Bhattacharyya et al. 2013).

It is becoming apparent that alterations in the lipid balance and protein content of lipid rafts is a key feature of neuroinflammation, neurodegeneration and ageing. Specifically, increases in the activity of the SFA palmitate, lead to increased post-translational protein modifications which result in increased protein targeting to lipid rafts. PUFAs can assist in disrupting excess age-related protein targeting to lipid rafts.

Further investigation into dietary lipid modifications to support Parkinson's patients is urgently required.

Alcohol, vitamin E and lipid rafts

Alcohol has been found to have beneficial properties at a low dosage, through its anti-inflammatory effect on lipid raft interaction with pathogens (Szabo et al. 2007). At higher intakes, alcohol has been linked with glial activation, neuroinflammation and cell death (Alfonso-Loeches et al. 2010). Furthermore, excessive alcohol consumption may lead to immune suppression and has been associated with increased risk of pneumonia and tuberculosis (Szabo et al. 2007).

α-Tocopherol is a form of vitamin E that has a high affinity for lipid rafts, where vulnerable PUFA rich phospholipids are in need of protection from lipid peroxidation. Some researchers have questioned whether α-tocopherol in lipid rafts could be viewed as *"an oar in the lifeboat?"* (Lemaire-Ewing et al. 2010). Furthermore, α-tocopherol can help prevent the incorporation of highly damaging cholesterol oxides into lipid rafts (Royer et al. 2009).

The Light Side of Oestrogen and Parkinson's Disease

Oestrogens form a group of hormones which act on much more than just reproductive tissue. In both men and women, oestrogens act as neuroprotective compounds. Oestradiol, in particular, acts as a brain-derived neuroprotective factor and oestrogen receptors act to protect the nervous system from neurodegenerative disease and cognitive decline (Arevalo et al. 2015).

In studies it has been observed that female laboratory animals have both higher dopamine synthesis and turnover during periods of rising oestrogen levels. In women with Parkinson's disease, oestrogen administration can lessen the severity of symptoms and may explain why men are more susceptible to the disease (Leranth et al. 2000). Moreover, it has been found that there is a 68% increase in the risk of Parkinson's disease if a woman undergoes oophorectomy before menopause (Marras & Saunders-Pullman 2014).

During ageing there are many negative alterations to brain chemistry which may predispose the brain to Parkinson's disease. Increases in the activity of monoamine oxidase, calcium dysregulation, DNA damage, lipid peroxidation and protein oxidation are all factors which can play a contributory role in Parkinson's disease. Oestradiol treatment in female rats has been found almost to normalise many of these age-related alterations in brain chemistry (Kumar et al. 2015).

Phytoestrogens are neuroprotective

The polyphenols resveratrol and quercetin act as phytoestrogens. Although both compounds are not as hormonally active as oestrogens, they have nevertheless been shown to be neuroprotective in cell-based models of Parkinson's disease (Gélinas & Martinoli 2002).

Genistein from soy products and ginsenoside Rg1 derived from American ginseng, are both phytoestrogens which have been found to have potential neuroprotective properties in Parkinson's disease (Wang et al. 2005); (Hwang & Jeong 2010).

The Dark Side of Oestrogen and Dopamine Metabolites

Oestrogen and dopamine have both light and dark sides to their biochemistry, and therefore have to be treated with care and consideration, especially when prescribed or supplemented. They are both essential for health, yet their metabolism can produce genotoxic metabolites.

Oestrogen and dopamine can undergo hydroxylation to form catechol quinones. Oestrogen can be metabolised to catechol oestrogen quinone, and dopamine (a catecholamine) to dopamine quinone. Catechol quinones can form unstable depurinating adducts on DNA, leaving DNA vulnerable to damaging transformations. N-acetylcysteine, resveratrol, and to lesser extent α-lipoic acid and melatonin, have all shown potential to help prevent the formation of depurinating DNA adducts (Zahid et al. 2011).

Quinones and cancer

Catechol oestrogen quinones may play a role in breast and prostate cancer initiation and dopamine quinones have been associated with Parkinson's disease and neurodegeneration. Additionally, there is some evidence that catechol oestrogen quinones may also be neurotoxic. The 4-hydroxylation of oestrogens has been shown to form the most unstable and damaging DNA adducts (Gaikwad et al. 2011).

Cancer is generally less prevalent in Parkinson's disease patients, with the exception of prostate cancer, breast cancer and malignant melanoma (Rugbjerg et al. 2012); (Kareus et al. 2012), reinforcing the idea that these particular cancers may have some metabolic pathways in common with Parkinson's disease. Moreover, research into prostate cancer and malignant melanoma is finding that faulty oestrogen metabolism is playing an increasingly important role in the progression of these cancers (Lawrence et al. 2015); (Janik et al. 2014).

Quinone metabolism - COMT, N-acetylcysteine, glutathione and resveratrol

Methylation of dopamine and catechol oestrogens by the enzyme COMT (catechol-O-methyltransferase) can assist in preventing toxic adduct formation and metal-derived ROS generation (Zhu 2002); (Cavalieri et al. 2002); (Meiser et al. 2013).

As mentioned above, N-acetylcysteine and resveratrol are helpful in the prevention of catechol quinone formation. N-acetylcysteine can help to raise glutathione levels to enable detoxification of quinones (Meiser et al. 2013), and resveratrol can reduce the activity of CYP1B1, the enzyme which induces the 4-hydroxylation of oestrogen (Guengerich et al. 2003).

Quinone metabolism - NQO1 (NAD(P)H:quinone acceptor oxidoreductase 1)

The enzyme NQO1 (NAD(P)H:quinone acceptor oxidoreductase 1) is an important enzyme which acts to reduce and deactivate quinones, thereby helping to prevent oxidative stress and the depletion of thiols, such as the amino acid cysteine. The hydrocarbon benzene is more toxic to DNA when NQO1 activity is low.

NQO1 is able to maintain the important antioxidants CoQ10 and vitamin E in their active state as both antioxidants have quinone properties; CoQ10 is also known as ubiquinone and vitamin E forms a vitamin E quinone when oxidised (Dowd & Zheng 1995); (Dinkova-Kostova & Talalay 2010) .

NQO1 expression has been observed to be raised in the substantia nigra of patients with Parkinson's disease, probably due to the increased presence of quinone derivatives of dopamine (Dinkova-Kostova & Talalay 2010).

NQO1 can be induced by the transcription factor Nrf2

NQO1 can be induced by the transcription factor Nrf2 (nuclear factor erythroid 2–related factor 2) acting in concert with nuclear antioxidant response elements (Dinkova-Kostova & Talalay 2010). In addition to NQO1, Nrf2 can also increase the expression of many glutathione related enzymes, nerve growth factor, brain-derived neurotrophic factor, calcium-binding proteins, ferritin and helps support mitochondrial biogenesis (Tufekci et al. 2011). Furthermore, Nrf2 activation may help reduce the expression of inflammatory enzymes such as cyclooxygenase-2 (COX-2) and inducible nitric oxide synthase (iNOS) (Thomas & Beal 2007).

Many plant compounds can help induce Nrf2, including epigallocatechin-3-gallate from green tea, cinnamon, wasabi, sulforaphane from cruciferous vegetables, resveratrol from grapes, curcumin, lycopene and sulphur compounds from garlic (Tufekci et al. 2011); (Carmona-Ramírez et al. 2012).

In laboratory mice, the loss of Nrf2 expression resulted in neuronal death, due to excess oxidative stress and mitochondrial dysfunction. The activation of Nrf2 resulted in protection from neurodegeneration in mouse models of Parkinson's disease (Thomas & Beal 2007).

Many plant-derived antioxidants exert their protective effect by having both pro-oxidant and antioxidant properties

Paradoxically, many plant-derived antioxidants may exert their protective effect by having both pro-oxidant and antioxidant properties. Curcumin, and many other polyphenols, have been reported to activate Nrf2 and endogenous antioxidant gene transcription via the generation of ROS, such as hydrogen peroxide (Sandur et al. 2007); (Surh 2012).

Therefore, it may be that plant polyphenol activation of endogenous antioxidants, via generation of small amounts of ROS, provides a longer-lasting benefit to cells than the direct antioxidant activity that these natural compounds provide.

COMT relies on methylation to metabolise dopamine

To detoxify catechols (such as dopamine), COMT relies on the methyl donor SAM (S-adenosylmethionine). Increased levels of homocysteine may indicate a deficiency in SAM co-factors, or increased usage of SAM, potentially undermining COMT function. S-adenosylhomocysteine can also provide negative feedback to inhibit COMT (Müller 2009); (Goodman 2001).

Leptin and conjugated equine oestrogens are further inhibitors of COMT, possibly implicating insulin resistance, type II diabetes and some HRT formulas in depurinating DNA adduct formation (Habib et al. 2015); (Yao et al. 2003). To ensure the correct operation of the methylation cycle and COMT, an adequate supply of co-factors, such as active folate, B12, B6 and magnesium is essential.

In Parkinson's disease, COMT activity may not be entirely beneficial and can be problematic in some circumstances. During Levodopa therapy COMT metabolises a proportion of Levodopa to toxic 3-O-methyldopa. (Müller 2009).

Levodopa therapy may result in an increased activity of COMT and a higher demand for methyl donor SAM. This may lead to depletion in SAM co-factors and therefore an increased risk of hyperhomocysteinaemia and related neurological and vascular effects (Müller 2009).

It has been observed that supplementation of SAM can exacerbate the symptoms of Parkinson's disease (Charlton & Mack 1994) since SAM supplementation may lead to co-factor depletion and an increase in homocysteine, in a similar way to L-DOPA therapy-related homocysteine increase. Moreover, homocysteine may act as a dopamine D2 receptor antagonist, potentially undermining the neuroprotective properties of this receptor (Agnati et al. 2006); (Ferrari-Toninelli et al. 2008).

COMT inhibition may increase neurotoxicity

COMT inhibition can help protect against hyperhomocysteinaemia, but may increase the level of genotoxic catechol oestrogen quinones and dopamine quinones. In addition, COMT inhibition within the central nervous system has been linked to increased ROS formation and the production of neurotoxic N-methylated tetrahydroisoquinolines.

N-methylated tetrahydroisoquinolines have been found to induce Parkinson's disease and are also seen in the cerebrospinal fluid and plasma of Parkinson's disease patients undergoing long term L-DOPA therapy (Müller 2009). In cell-based studies, dopamine loss triggered by tetrahydroisoquinolines was reversed by the antioxidant N-acetylcysteine (Surh & Kim 2010).

One type of tetrahydroisoquinoline is THP (tetrahydropapaveroline). THP is formed through the condensation of dopamine with its aldehyde metabolite, DOPAL. THP has been observed to inhibit the rate-limiting enzyme for dopamine synthesis, tyrosine hydroxylase, and has also been found to undermine mitochondrial function (Surh & Kim 2010).

During L-DOPA therapy, increasing availability of both dopamine and DOPAL are thought to be responsible for the rise in neurotoxic THP levels detected in the brain and urine of Parkinson's patients. Alcoholism can also lead to increases in THP and may be one of the reasons why alcohol abuse can lead to neurotoxicity (Surh & Kim 2010).

Plant polyphenol induction of Nrf2 may prove to be protective against THP, as Nrf2-linked expression of the enzyme haeme oxygenase (HO-1) has been observed in vitro to block THP mediated cell death (Surh & Kim 2010).

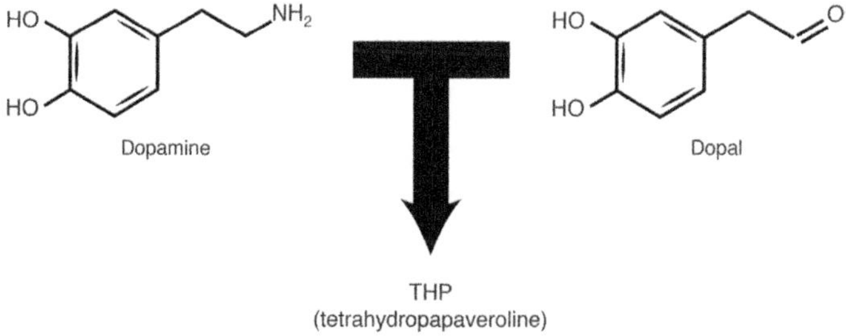

Dopamine → Dopal

THP
(tetrahydropapaveroline)

Dopamine condensation with DOPAL forms a neurotoxin called THP (tetrahydropapaveroline)

Microglia

Microglia are the resident macrophages of the brain and spinal cord and constitute approximately 10% of CNS cells. Under normal circumstances, microglia provide immune surveillance, acting as protectors against neurological disease (Aguzzi et al. 2013). If chronically activated, microglia can be drivers of neuroinflammation and, potentially, dopaminergic neuronal apoptosis. Resting microglia can become activated through inflammation or trauma, leading them to produce neurotoxic factors such as nitric oxide, peroxynitrite, superoxide, hydrogen peroxide and cytokines.

Microglial Activation and Parkinson's disease

Microglial neurotoxic factors can result in dopaminergic neuronal damage, eventually leading to the production and release of α-synuclein and neuromelanin. α-Synuclein and neuromelanin can, in turn, reactivate microglia, in a self-perpetuating cycle known as reactive microgliosis (Block et al. 2007).

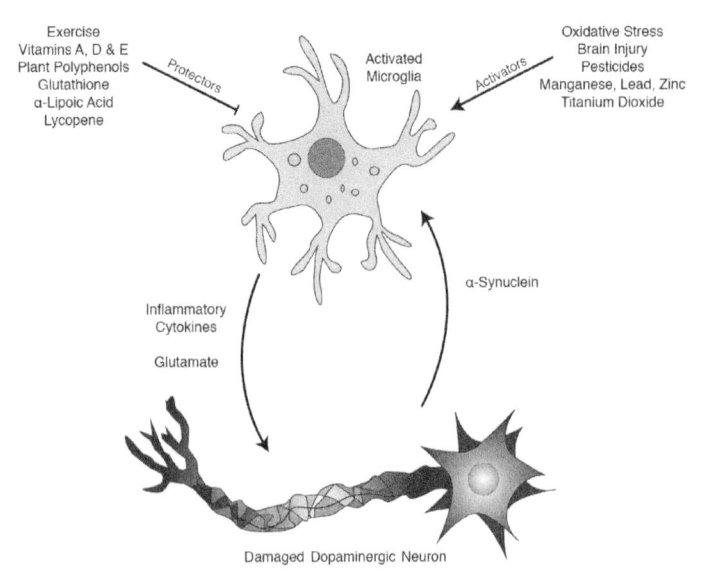

Activated microglia produce neurotoxic factors which can result in dopaminergic neuronal damage.

Metals, Toxic Exposure and Pesticides

The metal ion manganese mediates increased nitric oxide and inflammatory cytokine expression from activated microglia (Filipov & Dodd 2012). Manganese toxicity can lead to a condition known as manganism, which displays symptoms very similar to Parkinson's disease (Bourassa & Miller 2012).

Additionally, lead (Liu et al. 2012), titanium dioxide (Long et al. 2006) and zinc (Kauppinen et al. 2008) have all been found to be microglial activators.

There is an increased risk of Parkinson's disease for people exposed to the environmental toxins MPTP (1-methyl-4-phenyl-1,2,3,6-tetrahydropyridine), paraquat and rotenone.

These toxins have been found to increase oxidative stress in cell and animal models, leading to glial cell activation and dopaminergic neuron death (Miller et al. 2009).

Inflammation

Confirming the association with inflammation and Parkinson's disease, several studies have found a dramatic reduction in disease occurrence with regular users of NSAIDs, such as ibuprofen (Liu 2006).

The jury is out on whether ibuprofen would be of benefit to people presently suffering from Parkinson's disease, since the risk of gastrointestinal upset would have to be weighed against any benefits.

Hyperacetylation of the inflammatory transcription factor NF-kB can lead to microglial activation and the production of inflammatory cytokines (Pais et al. 2013).

The sirtuin SIRT2 is a deacetylase that may deacetylate NF-kB and decrease the transcription factor's activity, thereby helping to protect neurons from damaging inflammation. Some researchers have urged caution in up-regulating SIRT2 as SIRT2 inhibition may protect neurons exposed to α-synuclein (Pais et al. 2013).

Glutamate and Excitotoxicity

Activated microglia increase the synthesis of the excitotoxin glutamate via up-regulation of the enzyme glutaminase (Thomas et al. 2014).

Manganese disrupts the transport of both glutamine and glutamate which may be the mechanism behind manganese-induced neurotoxicity (Rajendram et al. 2015). Supplementation with glutamine and manganese should therefore be avoided in neurodegenerative diseases.

During oxidative stress, microglia can become a source of excitotoxic glutamate, with the potential to damage neurons.

Microglia increase glutathione synthesis during oxidative stress and require increased availability of the amino acid cysteine to support synthesis. Microglia import cysteine, in its oxidised form cystine, in exchange for the export of glutamate via the xc- cystine-glutamate exchanger.

Under normal conditions, glutamate is re-imported into the cytosol, but, during oxidative stress, re-import is inhibited, leaving excess extracellular excitotoxic glutamate available for neuronal uptake. Failure to re-import glutamate can further increase oxidative stress as glutamate is required to synthesise glutathione, alongside cysteine (reduced from cystine) and glycine (Mcbean 2012); (Barger & Basile 2001); (Porcheray et al. 2006).

Oxidative stress-induced inhibition of amino acid transporters can potentially be reversed by the antioxidant NAC. NAC's membrane permeability allows it to cross into cells without a transporter, where it can help reduce oxidative stress and also act as a precursor to glutathione synthesis. NAC has also been found to increase glutathione in dopaminergic neurons (Aoyama et al. 2008).

Nutrition and Microglia

Glutathione is a vital antioxidant which helps to maintain microglia in a resting inactive state. Microglia contain 78% more glutathione than can be found within neurons, and, via redox control, glutathione acts to raise the threshold of microglial activation.

Induction of iNOS can reduce microglial glutathione by approximately 40% (Rojo et al. 2014); (Hirrlinger et al. 2000). α-Lipoic acid is another neuroprotective antioxidant which can help protect microglial and dopaminergic cells from toxicity and oxidative stress (Muhamad Noor Alfarizal Kamarudin 2014).

Even though glutathione may be essential to support microglia function, it may be wise to be cautious regarding protocols aimed at raising glutathione. This is because, under certain circumstances, glutathione can increase the production of superoxide within lipid rafts of activated microglia (Faustino et al. 2011). Additionally, the metal ions manganese and zinc may activate microglia (Filipov & Dodd 2012); (Kauppinen et al. 2008).

Lycopene (Hsiao et al. 2004), apigenin & luteolin (Rezai-Zadeh et al. 2008), hyperforin (Lee et al. 2014), blueberry extract (Carey et al. 2013), bromelain (Habashi et al. 2012), 3,3'-diindolylmethane, (Kim et al. 2014), kaempferol, (Calderón-Montaño et al. 2011), curcumin, green tea, resveratrol, ginseng (Choi et al. 2011) and chrysanthemum indicum (Kim et al. 2011), are all plant-derived compounds that have been found to suppress microglial activation, in human, animal or in vitro studies.

Polyphenols from crowberry and bilberry have been shown to offer some degree of regeneration to the dopaminergic system (Rehnmark & Strömberg 2012).

It may also be worthwhile looking at methods to modify microglia phenotype from inflammatory M1 to neuroprotective M2 (Faustino et al. 2011). A deficiency of omega-3 PUFAs in developing animals leads to an inflammatory microglial phenotype (Madore et al. 2014). The transcription factor Nrf2 can upregulate endogenous antioxidant production and may help protect microglia from expressing an inflammatory phenotype (Rojo et al. 2010). Many of the polyphenols and natural compounds listed above are activators of Nrf2.

9-cis-retinoic acid is a natural derivative of vitamin A. 9-cis-retinoic acid has been observed to be a powerful suppressor of nitric oxide and inflammatory cytokines by microglia (Xu & Drew 2006). Interestingly, in Parkinson's disease, there is a deficiency in retinaldehyde dehydrogenase 1 (RALDH1), the enzyme necessary to synthesise retinoic acid (Nolan et al. 2013). The deficiency in RALDH1 parallels the deficiency in ALDH, another aldehyde dehydrogenase, and the enzyme required to detoxify the toxic dopamine metabolite, DOPAL.

Retinoic acid can suppress microglial activation, nitric oxide and inflammatory cytokine synthesis. Conversely, microglial activation can accelerate the degradation of retinoic acid (Hellmann-Regen et al. 2013), meaning that retinoic acid is an essential compound in protecting the CNS from inflammation. Retinoic acid is a vital compound for assisting the CNS in the repair and regeneration of neurons (Maden 2007).

Vitamin E has also been shown to have a suppressive effect on microglial activation in a similar way to retinoic acid (Li et al. 2001). Researchers have found that insufficient transport of vitamin E into the CNS can lead to neurodegeneration due to increases in oxidative stress (Yokota et al. 2001).

Benfotiamine is a synthetic, fat-soluble form of vitamin B1. Benfotiamine has been found to restore the shape and behaviour of activated microglia to that of inactive, non-stimulated microglia. In addition, benfotiamine decreased the expression of inflammatory mediators such as: inducible nitric oxide synthase (iNOS), cyclooxygenase-2 (COX-2) and inflammatory cytokines (Bozic et al. 2015).

Glial cell line-derived neurotrophic factor (GDNF) is a neurotrophic factor which is protective and restorative for dopaminergic neurons. 1,25-dihydroxyvitamin D3 (vitamin D3) can increase the activity of GDNF and protect against toxicity in animal models of Parkinson's disease (Wang et al. 2001).

Exercise has been proven to reduce neuroinflammation and microglial activation in laboratory mice with Parkinson's disease. Exercise is also thought to increase the regeneration of neurons through up-regulation of brain-derived neurotrophic factor (BDNF) (Jensen & Yong 2014).

Blood-Brain Barrier and Neurovascular Unit

The blood-brain barrier is constructed from endothelial cells bound together with tight junctions which maintain the barrier's integrity. The blood-brain barrier restricts the entry of blood-borne particles, yet allows the passage in of vital nutrients, and safe removal of waste products out of the brain.

The blood-brain barrier does not operate in isolation because it closely interacts with glial cells (brain immune cells) and neurons to form a '*neurovascular unit*'. The microenvironment maintained by the blood-brain barrier, and its interactions within the neurovascular unit, provide a stable environment for neuronal signalling (Abbott et al. 2006).

In Parkinson's disease, many studies have shown increased blood-brain barrier disruption associated with the condition. Increased inflammatory cytokine expression, such as interleukin 1 and TNF alpha, have been associated with neuroinflammation, and are likely to play a major role in blood-brain barrier permeability (Cabezas et al. 2014).

Disruption of the blood-brain barrier may allow peripheral inflammatory mediators and environmental toxins, such as pesticides, to cross more easily into the CNS and damage dopaminergic neurons.

Disruptors of the BBB

Inflammation

Monocyte chemoattractant protein-1 (MCP1) is a chemokine found to be up-regulated during inflammation. MCP1 has the ability to compromise the blood-brain barrier, resulting in excitotoxicity and the activation and migration of microglia (Yao & Tsirka 2014). MCP1 may be a useful blood marker for a patient's potential for a compromised blood-brain barrier.

Aluminium

Aluminium in the form of manufactured aluminium oxide nanoparticles, has been observed to decrease the expression of tight junction proteins, required to maintain the integrity of the blood-brain barrier. The mechanism of aluminium toxicity to the blood-brain barrier is thought to be via mitochondrial dysfunction within brain microvascular endothelial cells (Chen et al. 2008).

Reactive Oxygen Species

Reactive oxygen species (ROS) have been associated with the disruption of blood-brain barrier tight junction proteins (Schreibelt et al. 2007). The oxygen radical superoxide is a primary suspect linked to blood-brain barrier permeability, due to findings that the over-expression of the enzyme superoxide dismutase (SOD) may protect blood-brain barrier integrity (Schreibelt et al. 2007). Furthermore, the superoxide radical had been found to be the main reactive oxygen species involved in vascular permeability when the brain is exposed to cold temperatures (Yang & Rosenberg 2011).

It is of interest that motor neurone disease has been linked to mutant forms of SOD which are associated with decreased tight junction protein expression and increased permeability of the blood-spinal cord barrier (Zhong et al. 2008).

Zinc, Copper and Manganese

The trace minerals copper, zinc and manganese are co-factors required for two isoforms of superoxide dismutase (Keen et al. 1980). However, these trace minerals have also been observed to produce negative effects in relation to neuroinflammatory disease (Kauppinen et al. 2008); (Filipov & Dodd 2012); (Viles 2012).

Matrix metalloproteinases (MMPs) are a group of zinc-dependent enzymes associated with the breakdown of the blood-brain barrier. Endothelial cells of the blood-brain barrier exposed to the superoxide radical are thought to be compromised due to superoxide radical activation of MMPs (Gasche et al. 2001). Frustratingly, therefore, zinc may be implicated in both protecting and damaging the blood-brain barrier as a result of its role as a cofactor in superoxide dismutase and MMPs.

Obesity and Collagen Degradation

Obesity may lead to increases in blood-brain barrier permeability due its association with systemic inflammation, increases in vascular oxidative stress and MMP activation (McColl et al. 2010).

Neutrophils are a type of immune cell known to secrete MMP-9 and have been associated with blood-brain barrier permeability, in part due to collagen degradation by MMP-9 (Rosell et al. 2008). Furthermore, circulating neutrophils have been shown to be sources of high levels of oxidative stress in neurodegenerative diseases such as Parkinson's disease (Vitte et al. 2004).

The amino acid taurine can be chlorinated in the cytosol of neutrophils to form taurine chloramine. Taurine chloramine can decrease the production of nitric oxide, prostaglandin E2 and inflammatory cytokines to help dampen the tissue-damaging effects of neutrophils and macrophages (Marcinkiewicz et al. 1998).

Alcohol

Oxidative stress associated with the metabolism of alcohol can undermine blood-brain barrier integrity, leading to the migration of monocytes into the brain. The enzyme CYP2E1, induced during alcohol detoxification, increases ROS generation in the brain and is likely to play a role in alcohol consumption increasing blood-brain barrier permeability (Haorah et al. 2005).

Acetaldehyde, produced during alcohol metabolism, is a substrate for the enzyme aldehyde dehydrogenase. Aldehyde dehydrogenase is also an important enzyme for dopamine detoxification as its toxic by-product DOPAL is a substrate for aldehyde dehydrogenase. It is possible therefore, that alcohol may undermine the safe detoxification of dopamine.

Food Allergy, Histamine and Psychological Stress

Histamine produced via the activation of mast cells can lead to increased blood-brain barrier permeability. Food allergy triggers one mechanism which raises blood histamine levels, and psychological stress enables another.

Psychological stress results in increased mast cell degranulation and histamine release at the blood-brain barrier via the activation of corticotropin-releasing hormone (CRH) (Theoharides & Zhang 2011).

The effects of food allergy may be exacerbated in Parkinson's patients by increased immunoglobulin sensitivity due to excess palmitoylation within lipid rafts (Simons & Toomre 2000). Palmitoylation occurs when the saturated fat palmitate binds to proteins and alters their behaviour. The source of palmitate can be dietary or synthesised internally during inflammation, insulin resistance or as the result of a highly calorific meal.

The consumption of wheat and other gluten/gliadin containing foods has long been known to increase the permeability of the intestinal epithelium, via an increase in expression of the tight junction disrupting protein zonulin. More recently, zonulin has also been observed to increase the permeability of extraintestinal epithelial and endothelial tissue, including the blood-brain barrier (Fasano 2011).

Transepithelial Electrical Resistance (TEER)

Many other foods and food components can modify the permeability of the intestinal epithelium by modifying the transepithelial electrical resistance (TEER). A decrease in TEER can lead to increased epithelial permeability and maintaining TEER can help keep the integrity of the intestinal epithelium intact.

The spices paprika and cayenne pepper and many dietary fats can lead to decreases in TEER. Nutmeg, bay leaf, black pepper, quercetin, star anise, black tea, the probiotics L. plantarum and Bifidobacterium infantis have all been reported to increase TEER (Ulluwishewa et al. 2011). It is possible that the blood-brain barrier would also benefit from the above foods, bacteria and compounds. This is because the blood-brain barrier is dependent on a high TEER value to maintain its barrier integrity (Wilhelm et al. 2011).

Mannitol

Mannitol, a sugar alcohol or polyol found in many plants, is a disruptor of the blood-brain barrier but, paradoxically, may have some benefits for Parkinson's disease patients.

Mannitol causes osmotic shrinkage of endothelial cells within the blood-brain barrier, allowing the tight junctions to become more permeable. This property of mannitol makes it useful for use in combination with drugs targeted to the brain, to enable more of a dose to reach the CNS.

Furthermore, mannitol has properties that may protect α-synuclein from misfolding and aggregate formation (Shaltiel-Karyo et al. 2013). It may be wise to urge caution with the use of mannitol as a therapeutic agent for Parkinson's disease until further research confirms the above positive findings. The potential risk of increasing neuroinflammation, resulting from monocyte and environmental toxin infiltration, cannot be dismissed.

Nutrition and the blood-brain barrier

Ascorbate has been observed to offer some degree of protection for the integrity of the blood-brain barrier (Cabezas et al. 2014). Caffeine has also been reported to guard against blood-brain barrier leakage (Chen et al. 2010).

Vitamin D status is inversely associated with the activity of the blood-brain barrier degrading matrix metalloproteinase MMP-9 (Wasse et al. 2011).

The dipeptide carnosine can help protect superoxide dismutase (SOD) from fragmentation caused by hydroxyl radicals produced from the interaction of Cu/Zn-SOD and hydrogen peroxide (Choi et al. 1999). In addition to increasing plasma levels of Cu/Zn-SOD, carnosine can also increase the efficacy of L-DOPA therapy and can decrease lipid hydroperoxides (Choi et al. 1999). Furthermore, the quenching of hydroxyl radicals by carnosine can help to limit the oligomerization of α-synuclein (Kang & Kim 2003).

Olive oil polyphenols, resveratrol and quercetin have all been shown to inhibit MMP-9 in cultured endothelial cells (Scoditti et al. 2012).

Many studies have been reporting the beneficial effects of ingesting coffee and caffeine for both preventing Parkinson's disease and supporting patients with the disease. Amongst its many beneficial effects, caffeine has been found to improve the integrity of the blood-brain barrier by antagonising adenosine receptors. More specifically, it is the blocking or modulation of adenosine A2A and A2B receptors, which is considered to confer the benefit of caffeine to the blood-brain barrier (Chen et al. 2010).

Diamine oxidase is an enzyme which degrades histamine and is available in supplemental form. In relapsing-remitting Multiple Sclerosis, patients have been reported to have increased plasma histamine and low plasma diamine oxidase, potentially leading to increased blood-brain barrier permeability (Farokhi et al. 2014).

In Parkinson's disease, histamine metabolism is complicated by the depletion of histidine decarboxylase by the decarboxylase inhibitors carbidopa and benserazide, prescribed alongside L-DOPA medication (Hinz et al. 2014). It may be wise to measure plasma diamine oxidase in Parkinson's disease patients to ensure that they are able to metabolise histamine.

Summary

In summary, the integrity of the blood-brain barrier can be maintained by:

- Reducing inflammation
- Lowering psychological stress
- Avoiding allergens
- Abstaining from or lowering alcohol intake
- Removing wheat and gluten from diet
- Reducing ROS production and increasing SOD
- Identifying and removing aluminium sources
- Reducing factors associated with MMP activation.

The Glymphatic System

It has recently been discovered that the brain has its own lymphatic system – the glymphatic system. The designation glymphatic is derived from the words glia and lymphatic, as a type of glial cell called an astrocyte plays an essential role in this brain-cleansing mechanism.

Clearance of waste products and misfolded proteins from the brain is vital to help protect against neurodegenerative conditions such as Parkinson's and Alzheimer's disease. Research has suggested that around 65% of amyloid-β, the misfolded protein linked to Alzheimer's disease, is cleared via the glymphatic system.

It is highly likely that α-synuclein will be cleared in a similar manner. During sleep, the rate of waste product clearance from the brain is thought to double, highlighting the importance of adequate sleep in helping protect against neurodegeneration (Xie et al. 2013).

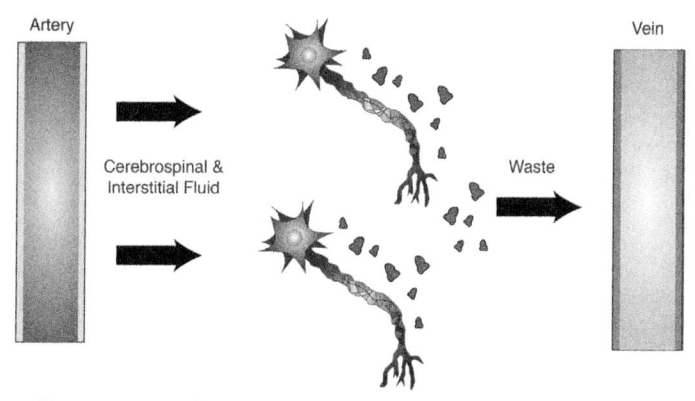

The clearance of waste and misfolded proteins from the brain occurs via the glymphatic system.

Metals, Ions and Neurotoxicity

Many metals and metal ions are toxic and of no biochemical value to human life. Many other metal ions are essential for biochemical reactions, yet simultaneously toxic and neurotoxic when conditions are unfavourable. Paradoxically, it is the instability of many metal ions that makes them effective as catalysts for redox reactions necessary for energy production, detoxification and neurotransmitter synthesis.

Metals such as mercury, arsenic, aluminium and lead are well-known toxic metals, but the dark sides of iron, calcium, manganese, copper and zinc are often overlooked. Parkinson's disease patients cannot afford to be complacent with these essential, yet potentially toxic metal ions (Hood & Skaar 2012); (Wright & Baccarelli 2007).

Metal Ions and Parkinson's disease

In Parkinson's disease, metal ions have been found to react with neuromelanin and α-synuclein. Furthermore, increased levels of iron, copper and zinc have been reported in human substantia nigra neurons.

Normally, neuromelanin has a high affinity for iron, with approximately 10-20% of substantia nigra iron bound to the compound. At higher iron concentrations, iron binds less securely to neuromelanin and increases the likelihood of free iron triggering toxic hydroxyl radical formation via the Fenton reaction (Bourassa & Miller 2012).

Tyrosine hydroxylase can be modified by dopamine quinones to form a quinoprotein linked with the reduction of iron and copper, contributing to oxygen radical formation in dopamine producing neurons (Bisaglia et al. 2013).

α-Synuclein is a protein which readily binds to metals. Iron, copper, aluminium and cobalt in vitro have been reported to accelerate the aggregation of α-synuclein from two weeks to just one day. Lewy bodies in the brain of Parkinson's disease patients contain a high level of aluminium, and diets high in iron have been found to increase the risk of Parkinson's disease (Lema Tomé et al. 2012).

α-Synuclein has a particularly high affinity for copper, with at least three binding sites found so far (Bourassa & Miller 2012). Aluminium readily binds to ATP, displacing the co-factor magnesium, leading to a disruption in energy production (Exley 2014).

Manganese can be neurotoxic

Manganese is a metal ion which displays neurotoxic effects via the activation of microglia. Expression of glial-derived nitric oxide and inflammatory cytokines, have been associated with apoptosis of substantia nigra neurons (Filipov & Dodd 2012).

Manganism is a Parkinson's-like disease caused by occupational exposure to manganese compounds. Manganese is a component of steel, leading to the possibility of increased manganese exposure for steelworkers and welders. It has been postulated, but not yet proven, that occupational exposure may lead to an earlier onset of Parkinson's disease in some manganese-exposed workers (McMillan 2005).

Parkinson's disease is associated with altered mitochondrial calcium

Altered mitochondrial calcium is thought to play an important role in the pathogenesis of Parkinson's disease. The endoplasmic reticulum (ER) acts as a cellular calcium store and a host site for the folding of proteins such as α-synuclein. ER stress leads to the activation of the unfolded protein response (UPR), calcium depletion and rapid calcium uptake by mitochondria.

Mitochondria assist in the control of cytosolic calcium by absorbing the ion and thereby keeping cytosolic calcium within normal limits. Excess cytosolic calcium plays a role in neuronal cell death triggered by glutamate induced excitotoxicity. Glutamate activates NMDA receptors to allow calcium influx into a cell.

Elevated cellular calcium can further activate the nitric oxide synthase enzymes nNOS and iNOS (Braidy et al. 2010). Both nNOS and iNOS are associated with α-synuclein aggregation, ER and mitochondrial dysfunction. Other potentially-damaging calcium-dependent enzymes are xanthine oxidase, monoamine oxidase A, phospholipase A2 and COX-2 (Seidl & Potashkin 2011).

The prevention of mitochondrial calcium overload and calcium-induced mitochondrial membrane collapse potential may form part of future interventions for many neurological diseases.

Titanium is damaging to the central nervous system

Titanium is a metal that has appeared in many new products in recent years; from sunscreen to skimmed milk to orthopaedic and dental implants. Titanium is generally recognised as safe for human exposure and consumption, but worryingly, an increasing number of studies are finding titanium dioxide nanoparticles to be damaging to the central nervous system.

Titanium dioxide nanoparticles can activate microglia (Long et al. 2006), known to be toxic to dopaminergic neurons, and can increase α-synuclein aggregation in vitro (Wu & Xie 2014). It is of concern that products not thought to contain titanium dioxide nanoparticles may nevertheless be a source.

Many samples of food-grade titanium dioxide (E171) have been found consist of roughly 20% nano-sized particles (Yang et al. 2014). Orthopaedic and dental implants may oxidise or undergo wear and tear which can subsequently lead to the formation of titanium oxides in the nanoparticle range (Skocaj et al. 2011).

Nutrition and Metal Ions

It is important for a Parkinson's disease patient to examine their diet and environment for all sources of toxic or reactive metals. Supplemental sources of metal ions or minerals may be safe for a healthy patient, but a Parkinson's disease patient must exercise caution, even if tests reveal an overt deficiency.

Ageing populations may display iron and calcium deficiencies, but Parkinson's patients should seek a second opinion if advised to take these metal ions as a supplement. Many health professionals may not be well-informed regarding the neurotoxicity of iron, calcium and other metal ions.

Citric acid can complex with aluminium and help prevent energy loss resulting from aluminium binding to, and inhibiting, ATP (Exley 2014). Frustratingly, though, aluminium citrate may accelerate aluminium transport to the brain (Nagasawa et al. 2005). Silicilic acid is another acid that can complex with, and inhibit, aluminium absorption and biological activity.

Aluminium can bind a thousand times more readily to ATP than magnesium, implying that evolution never designed life to deal with this toxic metal!

It is only in the last 100 years that the toxic aluminium 'genie' has been released from the bottle as the modern world found the means to release the metal from bauxite (Exley 2014).

Ageing leads to an increasing accumulation of aluminium in tissue, including the brain. Consumption of silicon-rich mineral waters has been found to reduce the body burden of aluminium (Davenward et al. 2013).

Ceruloplasmin is a copper and iron transport protein which can undergo modification by ROS, leading to the release of copper and an associated increase in α-synuclein aggregation. The dipeptide carnosine can help protect ceruloplasmin from damaging modifications (Kim et al. 2002).

Heat-shock Proteins and Chaperones

Unfrying an Egg!

A major characteristic of many neurodegenerative diseases is the highly damaging accumulation of misfolded protein. Parkinson's, Alzheimer's, Huntingdon's and Creutzfeldt-Jakob diseases have all been strongly associated with misfolded proteins as part of their pathogenesis. In the future, the secret to protecting against misfolded proteins and the refolding and removal of aggregates may be discovered through learning how to 'unfry' an egg!

The reason an egg white is 'white' after cooking is because heat denatures and misfolds the proteins within the egg. Experiments have shown that an egg can be effectively unfried with the use of proteins called 'chaperones'(Rozema & Gellman 1996); (Ben-Zvi & Goloubinoff 2001).

Understanding how to up-regulate the activity of chaperones and types of chaperone called 'heat-shock proteins' may be an important strategy to prevent the misfolding of α-synuclein and help in the disaggregation of aggregates.

The image of a denatured egg white gives a striking image of the problems occurring in the neural proteins of a Parkinson's disease patient.

Future strategies to support heat-shock proteins and chaperones

As the name suggests, heat-shock proteins are chaperones which are up-regulated as the heat increases around cells. This is a normal process that protects body proteins from denaturing or 'cooking' when exposed to high temperature.

An egg-white changes its appearance from clear to white, since the protein within the egg white starts to tangle and misfold when exposed to heat. In Parkinson's disease, the protein α-synuclein misfolds in a similar way, but it is neuroinflammation and exposure to excess reactive oxygen species which are largely responsible for misfolding and aggregation of the protein.

A study using laboratory animals seems to confirm the promise of heat-shock proteins as a way of protecting against α-synuclein aggregation. In the study, a virus was used to mediate overexpression of heat shock protein Hsp70. The authors found that:

"overexpression of Hsp70 holds significant potential as a disease-modulating therapeutic approach for Parkinson's disease" (Moloney et al. 2014)

Various methods of raising core body temperature have been employed to help with many health conditions and it does raise the possibility that the use of a sauna, foot spa, or a holiday in the sun may be able to activate the production of healing heat shock proteins.

The positive and negative aspects of valproic acid and lithium for neuroprotection

The drugs valproic acid and lithium, normally associated with epilepsy and bipolar disorder treatment respectively, may display some benefits in Parkinson's disease, but they are not without strong side effects. Both drugs have been reported to be neuroprotective via the activation of heat-shock protein 70 (Hsp70). Valproic acid may also help reduce the damaging activity of the pesticide Rotenone on complex I of the mitochondrial electron transport chain, as a result of its inhibition of apoptotic protein complexes (Pan et al. 2005).

Another benefit of lithium is its ability to reduce levels of lipid peroxides, such as 4-hydroxynonenal. 4-hydroxynonenal can form adducts with, and inhibit, vesicular monoamine transporter 2 (VMAT2), the transporter which sequesters dopamine into vesicles (Tan et al. 2012). It is possible, therefore, that lithium could protect against the toxicity of DOPAL by increasing the sequestration of dopamine and increasing the activity of ALDH (aldehyde dehydrogenase) enzymes.

Extreme caution must be exercised before considering valproic acid and lithium, since there have been reports of patients displaying Parkinsonism when prescribed these two drugs (Holroyd & Smith 1995); (Khwaja & Ranjan 2010), highlighting the need for further research to find appropriate dosages.

Valproic acid use at higher concentrations has been linked with significant depletion of antioxidant enzymes, increased lipid peroxidation and neurotoxicity (Chaudhary & Parvez 2012). Worryingly, valproic acid increases the activity of monoamine oxidase, the enzyme which degrades dopamine, and is often over-active in Parkinson's disease patients.

Long term lithium use is also not without potentially damaging side effects. The literature reports kidney dysfunction, hypothyroidism and an exacerbation or psoriasis in some patients (Albert et al. 2014).

Nutrition, heat-shock proteins and chaperones

Antarctic strains of the algae chlorella have been found to contain increased levels of heat-shock proteins, implying that thermal stress, whether through cold or heat, may increase their expression (Chankova et al. 2013). Another benefit of chlorella is that it contains the electron carrier plastoquinone, a quinone with greater anti-oxidant power than CoQ10 (Nakashima et al. 2014).

The stilbene resveratrol has been reported to up-regulate heat-shock proteins and protect motor neurons in laboratory animals (Han et al. 2012)

Resveratrol is an activator of SIRT1, an anti-ageing protein that deacetylates and enables heat-shock factor 1, a master regulator of heat-shock proteins (Han et al. 2012).

Therefore, resveratrol can be seen as an up-regulator of endogenous heat-shock proteins and chlorella a supplier of exogenous heat-shock proteins.

It could be that the consumption of plants from extreme environments may be beneficial in misfolded protein diseases such as Parkinson's.

Type 2 Diabetes and the Risk of Parkinson's Disease

Epidemiological studies have highlighted a potential link between type 2 diabetes and Parkinson's disease, indicating that patients with type 2 diabetes are 36% more likely to develop Parkinson's disease (Santiago & Potashkin 2013).

Worryingly, UK diabetes cases are predicted almost to double from the present 2.9 million to 5 million cases by 2025 (http://www.diabetes.org.uk/diabetes-in-the-uk-2014). This suggests that there could be a similar dramatic increase in Parkinson's disease cases. 60% of Parkinson's disease patients have faulty insulin signalling and are glucose intolerant (Santiago & Potashkin 2013).

Genes encoding the proteins Akt and DJ-1 can be altered in familial forms of both diabetes and Parkinson's disease, increasing susceptibility in both conditions. Furthermore, Parkinson's disease and diabetes share common cellular pathway dysregulation, including: mitochondrial dysfunction, ER stress, inflammation and vitamin D deficiency (Santiago & Potashkin 2013).

Insulin resistance, obesity and type 2 diabetes are all linked to over expression of fatty acid synthase (FASN), known as a 'lipogenic state' (Menendez et al. 2009).

A low-fat, high-carbohydrate diet may lead to increases in de novo palmitate synthesis, since the body is designed to store high glucose intakes as fat, via activation of FASN. Saturated fatty acids, such as palmitate, laurate and stearate, can increase CNS inflammatory cytokine synthesis (Hussain et al. 2013), with palmitate and stearate being found to be increased in Parkinson's disease brains (Kubo et al. 2015).

In animals fed an omega-3 PUFA-rich diet, gene expression of FASN was found to be suppressed (Teran-Garcia et al. 2007).

Misfolded proteins link Parkinson's disease with diabetes

At a deeper level, diabetes, in the same way as Parkinson's disease, has protein misfolding as part of its aetiology. Islet amyloid polypeptide (IAPP) or amylin is co-secreted with insulin from pancreatic β cells, working with both insulin and glucagon, to maintain glucose homeostasis (Ludvik et al. 1997).

It is thought that misfolded amylin may interact with both α-synuclein and amyloid-β, suggesting that amylin could play a role in Parkinson's and Alzheimer's disease respectively (Atsmon-Raz & Miller 2015); (Jackson et al. 2013). Conversely, misfolded α-synuclein may play a role in diabetes as α-synuclein has been detected in β cell potassium channels (Geng et al. 2011) The insulin-degrading enzyme (IDE) degrades not only insulin but also amyloid proteins such as α-synuclein (Steneberg et al. 2013). IDE is a zinc-dependent enzyme which can be inhibited by copper (Grasso et al. 2011).

The insulin-degrading enzyme (IDE) forms complexes with α-synuclein monomers, protecting β cells from α-synuclein oligomer formation and impaired insulin secretion (Steneberg et al. 2013).

Could IDE therefore play an potential role in protecting dopaminergic neurons from misfolded α-synuclein?

Nutrition to help prevent insulin-resistance and type 2 diabetes

Insulin is a hormone released from pancreatic beta cells in response to increases in blood glucose, after ingestion of food. In a healthy diet, much of the nutrition required to support insulin action and blood sugar balance is contained within the food being consumed.

Modern diets, obesity and stressors may lead to a depletion in these synergistic nutrients. Fortunately, the supplementation of several nutrients may be able to ameliorate dietary deficiencies in order to support patients with insulin-resistance and type 2 diabetes (Via 2012); (García et al. 2009).

α-Lipoic acid is a natural thiol antioxidant which has been found to help protect against metabolic syndrome, diabetes and neurodegeneration (Gomes & Negrato 2014).

Magnesium is frequently deficient in type 2 diabetes, metabolic syndrome and insulin resistance. Magnesium is a co-factor in several enzymes associated with energy production and glucose metabolism; its deficiency is linked to glycated haemoglobin and poor insulin regulation (Barbagallo & Domínguez 2013).

Oily fish intake of approximately 80g per day has been found to reduce the risk of type 2 diabetes by 20% (Zhang et al. 2013).

Taurine is showing promise as a protective agent against many aspects of diabetes. Moreover, taurine can support mitochondrial electron transport and buffering of the mitochondrial matrix (Ito et al. 2012).

The polyphenols resveratrol and curcumin are found in fruit and the spice turmeric. Both of these polyphenols have been found to protect and enhance pancreatic β cell function (Rouse et al. 2014).

The Cytoskeleton and Neurodegeneration

The cytoskeleton is an intracellular structure composed of three types of protein filament, which enables a cell to maintain its shape, motility and internal organisation. The largest component is the microtubule, next is the intermediate filament, and the smallest is just the filament (Kapitein & Hoogenraad 2015).

The microtubule is constructed from polymers of the proteins α and β tubulin. Microtubules allow cargo, such as organelles, to be transported on microtubule tracks throughout a cell. In neurons, microtubules are essential for efficient mitochondrial energy production and delivery, due to the relatively long distances between the cell body and the synapse.

Mitochondria are attached to microtubules via protein motors which drive mitochondria to areas of energetic need within a neuron. The synapse of a neuron requires high levels of ATP for energy and is vulnerable when ATP levels drop significantly (Kapitein & Hoogenraad 2015).

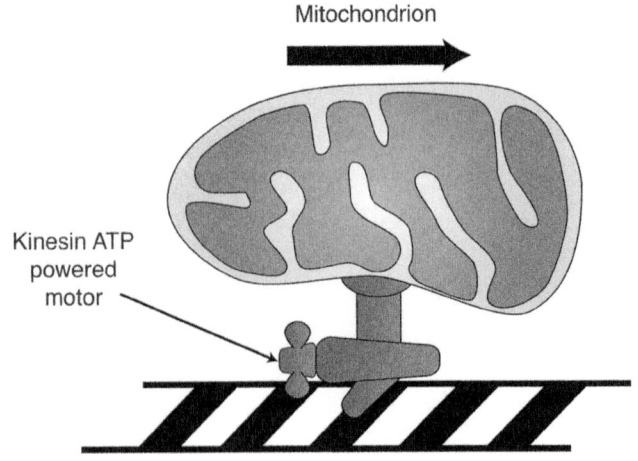

Organelles, such as mitochondria, travel along a neuron on cytoskeletal tracks (constructed of microtubules). Mitochondria are powered by ATP fuelled kinesin motors.

Filaments are constructed from the protein actin. It is the interaction of actin filaments and microtubules that is essential for the development of neuronal axons and dendrites. Neurodegenerative disease often begins with axonal degeneration; the fragmentation of microtubules being one of the first events to occur (Kapitein & Hoogenraad 2015).

Psychological Stress

Psychological stress has been found to have a negative impact on Parkinson's disease outcome, resulting both from observation and clinical studies. Exacerbation of microglial activation is one mechanism by which psychological stress may lead to dopaminergic neuronal death (de Pablos et al. 2014). Other studies have analysed the effects of psychological stress on stress hormone induction and microglial perturbation (Walker et al. 2013). Research into the effects of immobilisation stress are showing some very promising results.

Laboratory animals immobilised and restrained for several hours a day showed increased expression of tyrosine hydroxylase, tetrahydrobiopterin and dopamine along with raised lipid peroxidation, neuromelanin and oxidative damage to dopaminergic neurons (Kim et al. 2005). At a biochemical level, this study highlights the deleterious effect of over-stimulating dopaminergic neurons, a factor not currently addressed by many clinicians. At a psychological level, the reaction of an animal or person to the effects of inescapable stress, appears to play an important role in predisposing them to damage within the nigrostriatal system. It is damage within the nigrostriatal system which leads to Parkinson's disease.

In Parkinson's disease, psychological stress may lead to "freezing", where a person is left unable to walk for a short period of time. This effect may be triggered by negative thoughts, emotions and stress, but has been found to be effectively countered by relaxation and cognitive techniques (Macht & Ellgring 1999).

L-DOPA-induced Dyskinesias (LIDs)

L-DOPA (L-3,4-dihydroxyphenylalanine) - induced dyskinesias (LIDs) are abnormal or involuntary movements which appear in Parkinson's disease patients during L-DOPA therapy. After 5 years of L-DOPA therapy it is estimated that around 50% of patients will be experiencing LIDs (Mosharov et al. 2015).

The two main types of dyskinesia are chorea and dystonia. Chorea can be described as involuntary movement which displays itself in irregular patterns throughout the body. The name chorea is derived from the Greek word for 'dance' (Micheli & LeWitt 2014). Dystonia is defined as abnormal, involuntary muscle contractions which may result in repetitive postures, twisting or other movements (Albanese et al. 2013).

Types of L-DOPA-induced dyskinesias (LIDs)

"Peak-dose" dyskinesias are expressed when plasma levels of L-DOPA are at their highest. Peak-dose dyskinesias are choreic movements displayed as involuntary twitching or jerking, usually close to L-DOPA administration (Mosharov et al. 2015).

Diphasic dyskinesias occur at "on/off" phases of L-DOPA administration and can display as both chorea and dystonia (Fahn 2000).

"Off" dyskinesia is a dystonia that occurs when the effect of L-DOPA medication has diminished. This type of dystonia must not be confused with dystonia that is a signature of the Parkinson's disease process (Fahn 2000).

What causes LIDs?

One theory about the cause of LIDs is that there is presynaptic dysregulation of striatal dopaminergic neurons. With the progressive loss of dopaminergic neurons, it becomes increasingly difficult safely to store dopamine, associated with L-DOPA administration, in storage vesicles. The loss of storage vesicles is thought to result in high synaptic dopamine levels that correlate with "peak-dose" dyskinesias (Mosharov et al. 2015).

Another theory implicates striatal serotonergic neurons processing L-DOPA and releasing dopamine as a "false neurotransmitter". It has been shown that administering a serotonin agonist before a dose of L-DOPA can reduce the severity of LIDs (Politis et al. 2014).

Like dopaminergic neurons, serotonergic neurons also use the enzyme AADC (aromatic L-amino acid decarboxylase), but instead normally synthesise 5-HTP (5-hydroxytryptophan) rather than dopamine. This similarity in metabolism allows for the "false neurotransmission" effect in Parkinson's disease (Mosharov et al. 2015). In later stages of Parkinson's disease, it is thought that the majority of L-DOPA to dopamine synthesis occurs in striatal serotonergic neurons (Mosharov et al. 2015).

LIDs – The way forward

The peak-dose dyskinesia problem has led several drug companies to develop delivery systems to provide a lower dosage and a more constant supply of L-DOPA for Parkinson's disease patients. To this end, there are belt and patch pumps, inhalers, intestinal gel and 'accordion style' slow-release capsules, all being developed (Dolhun 2015).

Aromatic L-amino Acid Decarboxylase (AADC) Inhibitors and Vitamin B6 Deficiency

In 1975, L-DOPA began to be prescribed with an AADC inhibitor, to help reduce the nausea due to the peripheral conversion of L-DOPA to dopamine. Additionally, with less peripheral conversion of L-DOPA to dopamine, the drug combination allowed L-DOPA to be prescribed at much reduced dosages (Hinz et al. 2014).

AADC inhibitors and vitamin B6

A potential problem with AADC inhibitors is that they are not totally selective to the enzyme. Consequently, they can irreversibly inhibit not only AADC but vitamin B6, in its pyridoxal 5'-phosphate (PLP) form, and other PLP dependent enzymes (Daidone et al. 2012).

Over 300 enzymes require PLP for their function and thus PLP loss, via the action of AADC inhibitors, is likely to be far-reaching (Hinz et al. 2014). It might be that future interventions will have to balance the benefits of AADCs (in preventing nausea and increasing drug efficacy), against the negative effects of PLP depletion. Alternatively, developing a drug that exhibits selective inhibition of AADC would also help address the PLP depletion issue.

Serotonin, histamine and blood sugar are affected by AADC inhibitors

The conversion of L-DOPA to dopamine is not the only activity of AADC. The conversion of 5-Hydroxytryptophan (5-HTP) to serotonin, and histidine to histamine are also dependent on the enzyme. Histamine is an important regulator of dopamine in nigrostriatal neurons of the basal ganglia and histamine depletion may therefore be problematic (Clementi 2006).

The peripheral inhibition of AADC may also lead to hypoglycaemia, since AADC-dependent catecholamines are required to maintain glucose homeostasis during fasting (Arnoux et al. 2013).

L-DOPA and dopamine interrelationship with other neurotransmitters

In addition to the peripheral disruption of AADC-dependent amines and PLP-dependent enzymes by AADC inhibitors, L-DOPA itself may disrupt the balance of amino acids and neurotransmitters. L-DOPA and dopamine display a complex interrelationship with many neurotransmitters and amino acids (Hinz et al. 2014).

Biomarkers for Parkinson's Disease

A search for valid blood biomarkers for Parkinson's disease has uncovered two promising proteins, both with links to diabetes and insulin signalling. The mRNAs of Hepatocyte nuclear factor 4 alpha (*HNF4A*) and the polypyrimidine tract binding protein 1 (*PTBP1*) were shown to be respectively up-regulated and down-regulated in Parkinson's patients (Santiago & Potashkin 2015).

Blood plasma levels of phosphorylated and total α-synuclein may prove to be useful biomarkers in Parkinson's disease (Foulds et al. 2013).

Several gene variations have been identified as potential markers for familial cases of Parkinson's disease. These are the genes that encode for LRRK2 (leucine-rich repeat kinase 2), Parkin, DJ-1, PINK1 (PTEN-induced putative kinase 1) and α-synuclein, all with links to mitochondrial function (Sai et al. 2012). Familial cases of Parkinson's are very rare, with less than 5% of cases classified this way.

Sporadic Parkinson's disease constitutes the majority of Parkinson's disease cases, and now gene analysis for genes with a low penetrance may soon be possible for this Parkinson's disease classification. Examining whole genome gene expression enables researchers to compile data on vast numbers of genes, and whether they are under-expressed or over-expressed genes in Parkinson's disease cases, compared to controls (Lewis & Cookson 2012).

Tyrosine Kinase inhibition
A new hope from oncology

The non-receptor tyrosine kinase c-Abl has been reported to be activated during oxidative stress and in the dopaminergic pathways of Parkinson's disease patients. Furthermore, drug inhibition of c-Abl in animal models has been shown to reduce the damaging effects of the disease.

Non-receptor tyrosine kinase inhibitors are a class of drug developed for chronic myeloid leukaemia but they have also been showing great promise in Parkinson's and Alzheimer's disease research (Karuppagounder et al. 2014); (Imam et al. 2013).

Excess phosphorylation of proteins is problematic in Parkinson's disease

Excess phosphorylation of the proteins α-synuclein and parkin is a signature of Parkinson's disease. Phosphorylation of α-synuclein leads to increased aggregation of the protein. Phosphorylation of parkin results in its inactivation, leading to loss of parkin's neuroprotective function (Mahul-Mellier et al. 2014).

Parkin is an E3 ubiquitin ligase involved in the ubiquitination and proteosomal degradation of proteins. Parkin can help maintain the integrity of mitochondria by initiating the removal of old or dysfunctional organelles via mitophagy. Additionally, parkin can help prevent neuronal cell apoptosis by inhibiting the translocation of the proapoptotic protein Bax to mitochondria (Charan et al. 2014). Mutations in the *parkin* gene are associated with familial Parkinson's disease, with *parkin* gene mutations being the most common cause of young-onset Parkinson's disease (Abouhamdan et al. 2011).

c-Abl inhibitors can reduce the excitotoxicity of glutamate

In Parkinson's disease, some motor irregularities seen in the condition are caused by an imbalance between dopamine and glutamate in the striatum. Dopamine deficiency and c-Abl can both lead to excessive glutamate transmission. Studies have shown that this imbalance can be abrogated by c-Abl inhibitors, which suppress glutamate transmission in the striatum (Tanabe et al. 2014).

c-Abl inhibitors are showing promise in phase 1 drug trials

It can be seen from the above that excess c-Abl expression can lead to the loss of parkin activity, increased α-synuclein aggregation and motor irregularities in the striatum.

Pharmacological inhibition of c-Abl is potentially an effective way of addressing some key biochemical issues related to Parkinson's disease. Research into c-Abl inhibitors is ongoing, with results from phase 1 trials showing many positive outcomes.

Uric Acid – Friend or Foe?

Purines provide vital components for the nucleic acids RNA and DNA, and the energy carriers ATP, FADH2 and NADH. When purines break down in our metabolism, the resulting end-product is uric acid.

As a result of a quirk of evolution, humans and other great apes cannot degrade uric acid, since a gene mutation means that we no longer have the enzyme uricase (Johnson et al. 2005). As we shall see, this mutation is both a benefit and a curse!

Ideally, purine production and degradation should be in balance, with uric acid being cleared by the kidneys and bowel. Excess purine production, dietary consumption, kidney dysfunction or excess purine degradation can all lead to increased blood levels of uric acid.

Whether increased blood uric acid is problematic largely depends on the individual.

Uric acid is both a powerful antioxidant and, in its crystalline form, an extremely damaging inflammatory agent. As an antioxidant, uric acid is a highly efficient scavenger of reactive oxygen and nitrogen radicals, both of which play a major role in the pathology of Parkinson's disease (Pakpoor et al. 2015).

In crystalline form, uric acid (along with asbestos, cholesterol crystals and aluminium) is an activator of the inflammasome, a complex which drives inflammation. Increased blood uric acid is associated with gout, kidney stones, cardiovascular disease, hypertension and metabolic syndrome (Maiuolo et al. 2016).

The Benefits of Uric Acid for Parkinson's Disease

Dopamine binding to the dopamine transporter decreases as Parkinson's disease progresses. Uric acid can help maintain dopamine transporter binding, to help protect from disease progression (Moccia et al. 2015). Since dopamine transporter inhibitors are a class of drugs used in Parkinson's disease, it is essential to seek professional advice before supplementing any purine derivative.

In addition to a direct benefit in dopaminergic neurons, uric acid had been found to support many non-motor symptoms in Parkinson's disease. Higher uric acid levels have been associated with improved attention and memory, reduced cardiovascular events and improved sleep (Moccia et al. 2014). Interestingly, both low and high blood uric acid could potentially be implicated in cardiovascular disease.

Patients with Parkinson's disease, multiple sclerosis and motor neurone disease have been found to suffer from less gout than the general population (Pakpoor et al. 2015). One hypothesis regarding Parkinson's disease is that the pathology of the condition may be behind the lowered uric acid seen in patients (Sampat et al. 2016). This does suggest that Parkinson's disease patients may benefit from increased purine consumption, whilst taking every precaution to protect against uric acid crystal formation. Monitoring of safe blood uric acid levels, kidney function and markers for systemic inflammation is therefore essential.

Nutrition and uric acid

Researchers have experimented with raising blood and nervous system uric acid by supplementing inosine. Inosine is a nucleoside that readily degrades to uric acid. It was found that raising blood levels to around 7mg/dL was well tolerated by patients. Three participants did develop kidney stones during the study. Cardiovascular problems were equally found in inosine intervention patients and controls (Schwarzschild et al. 2014).

Diet has a profound effect on blood uric acid levels with large meals, alcohol, sugary drinks and fruit juice all increasing the risk of gout. Every meal containing meat increases the risk of gout by a staggering 21%. Body mass index is another factor which increases blood uric acid and gout risk. Milk and coffee consumption both increase the excretion of uric acid and therefore lessen gout risk. Vegetarians are the group most likely to have low blood uric acid levels due to dairy consumption and avoidance of animal purine sources (Nickolai & Kiss 2016); (Schmidt et al. 2013).

Surprisingly, vegans have high blood purine levels but without the associated increased risk of gout (Schmidt et al. 2013). Vegans often consume beans and pulses which are high in purine content. Although beans and pulses may be difficult for many people to tolerate, it does go to show that uric acid per se is not necessarily the issue; poor oxidant status, high BMI and an acidic metabolism, may all increase the chance of uric acid becoming an enemy rather than a very useful friend.

A ketogenic diet for neuroprotection

High saturated fat consumption is usually seen in a negative light but, strangely, eating more saturated fat can, in some cases, be beneficial. The key to this beneficial switch in fat metabolism is reliant on a very low carbohydrate intake, causing the liver to export compounds called ketones bodies. Ketones bodies or ketones are partially-metabolised molecules of fat which the liver cannot deal with. This is because the liver requires a small amount of carbohydrate to process fat. The liver's loss is the brain's gain, since the brain (along with muscle, kidneys and heart) can all use ketones for energy.

There have been many reports of the benefits of a diet that produces ketones (ketogenic diet) to help with Parkinson's disease, Alzheimer's disease and epilepsy. The positive and negative characteristics of ketone metabolism will be examined in this chapter.

Ketone metabolism

Acetoacetate, beta-hydroxybutyrate (β-OHB), and acetone are the three types of ketone body formed by the liver. The lungs can clear acetone, and it is the fruity odour of acetone on a person's breath that gives an indication that they are metabolising ketones.

Due to the inefficiency of long chain fatty acids (LCFA) metabolism, the classic ketogenic diet requires a 4:1 ratio of LCFAs to protein and carbohydrate making it a very difficult diet to adhere to.

LCFAs cannot enter the bloodstream or mitochondria without added assistance. LCFAs have to be carried by chylomicrons in the lymphatic system before entering general circulation. To enter mitochondria, LCFAs require carnitine to assist them in entering the mitochondrial matrix. The inefficient transport of LCFAs is further compounded by the many cycles of β-oxidation required to fully metabolise fatty acids (Branco et al. 2016).

Consumption of medium chain triglycerides (MCTs) can be a more palatable dietary intervention to raise blood ketone levels. Furthermore, because MCTs do not require chylomicrons or carnitine for their transport, they can enter the bloodstream and mitochondria more rapidly than LCFAs. The increased metabolic efficiency of MCTs means that a ketogenic diet on these fats allows for extra food choices, and therefore is more likely to have higher patient compliance (Branco et al. 2016).

Ketones and the brain

The brain cannot metabolise fat for energy, but it can utilise ketones. In fact, as the brain ages, it struggles to use glucose as a fuel but doesn't have the same difficulty with ketones (Masino et al. 2016). In Parkinson's disease, ketones have been shown to protect dopaminergic neurons from toxicity and maintain mitochondrial energy production, when there are defects in the electron transport chain (Paoli et al. 2014). In one trial, Parkinson's disease patients reported a 43% drop in disease markers whilst on a ketogenic diet.

A ketogenic diet has been found to increase the manufacture of new mitochondria, to increase glutathione levels and to improve oxygen efficiency (Dedkova & Blatter 2014). The benefits of a ketogenic diet in epilepsy could be due to ketones helping support dysfunctional mitochondria (Kim et al. 2015); (Branco et al. 2016). Therefore, ketones may be able to maintain neuronal ATP production, despite mitochondrial dysfunction.

The dangers of a ketogenic diet

Frustratingly, a ketogenic diet is far from the utopian diet that many purport it to be. Side effects are many, such as: Low magnesium and calcium, lethargy, cardiomyopathy, constipation, kidney stones, nausea, weight loss, reduced bone density, diarrhoea, hyperlipidaemia, vomiting, acidosis and gout (Branco et al. 2016); (Klein et al. 2014). In addition, a patient needs to be able to digest, absorb and metabolise fats fully, to gain any benefit. The digestion and absorption of many nutrients can be compromised in Parkinson's disease patients.

Excess blood ketones can lead to a dangerous condition called ketoacidosis. Ketoacidosis may occur in types 1 & 2 diabetes due to the loss of insulin or insulin sensitivity. If blood levels of ketones go above 3 mmol/L this is considered to put a patient at risk of ketoacidosis (Dhatariya & Savage 2013).

Nutritional ketosis for Parkinson's disease

For Parkinson's disease and neuroprotection, a lower level of blood ketones is utilised and is known as nutritional or dietary ketosis. Typically, blood levels of ketones will increase to between 1 and 2 mmol/L when on a nutritional ketosis diet (Pinckaers et al. 2016).

A Parkinson's disease patient (or, indeed, any patient) should seek full professional guidance and support if they wish to embark on a ketogenic diet. It is crucial that their blood ketones are monitored and maintained in the nutritional ketosis range. Blood ketones should not be allowed to increase to levels that are too high, putting the patient at risk of moving into ketoacidosis.

Can nutritional intervention help repair dopaminergic synapses?

An overview of brain regions involved in Parkinson's disease

Before discussing nutritional intervention to support dopaminergic synapses, it is probably wise to consider the area of the brain afflicted by Parkinson's disease.

Dopaminergic neurons of the substantia nigra pars compacta extend via the nigrostriatal pathway into the striatum of the basal ganglia. The loss of these dopaminergic neurons leads to a motor control deficit and results in the characteristic tremor observed in Parkinson's disease.

The names substantia nigra pars compacta, striatum and nigrostriatal pathway may all sound complex terms, but they are just simple labels for the brain regions or components being described.

Substantia nigra pars compacta can be easily translated to: compact region of black substance.

Striatum: describes the striped appearance of the nerve fibres when cross-sectioned (Purves et al. 2001).

Nigrostriatal pathway: describes the path dopaminergic neurons take from the substantia nigra to the striatum. i.e. a path from a black to a striped region!

The substantia nigra is a 'black substance' precisely because of the high levels of dopamine this area of the brain metabolises. As Parkinson's disease progresses, the region becomes pale in colour, since less dopamine is produced (Zecca et al. 2001).

In a similar way to the amino acid tyrosine, dopamine can be metabolised into the pigment melanin. Neuromelanin is the type of melanin found within the substantia nigra which gives the region its dark appearance.

It is interesting how simple terms can appear complicated when translated into Latin! Now that the terms are easier to understand it will hopefully make more sense when discussing the areas of the brain involved in Parkinson's disease.

Of central importance in Parkinson's disease is the connection between the nigrostriatal dopaminergic neurons and the striatum in maintaining nervous system control of motor function.

Synapses from the nigrostriatal neurons have to connect with striatum dendrites to be able to complete the motor circuits of the basal ganglia. As Parkinson's disease progresses, there is a steady decline in these striatal synapse to dendrite connections.

Three nutrients to help restore dopaminergic synapses

There have been some potentially ground-breaking discoveries in animal models of Parkinson's disease in relation to synapse integrity. The extremely promising research has discovered that feeding animals with synaptic precursor nutrients may help improve failing dopaminergic transmission. The nutrients were found to work by supporting synaptic terminals and dendritic spines, where nigrostriatal neurons interconnect with the striatum (Cansev et al. 2008).

The three key nutrients found to improve synaptic function were DHA, choline and uridine (as uridine monophosphate). If this research could be translated to Parkinson's disease patients, the authors of the study suggest there may be as much as a 15-25% increase in synaptic function. Bearing in mind that Parkinson's disease symptoms appear after a 70-80% loss of dopaminergic neurons (Cansev et al. 2008), this nutritional intervention may make a small but significant difference.

Instead of supplementing phosphatides (phospholipids) alone, supplementing the precursor nutrients can allow for the synthesis of the whole gamut of phosphatides. This includes: phosphatidylcholine, phosphatidylethanolamine, phosphatidylserine, phosphatidylinositol and sphingomyelin (Cansev et al. 2008).

An additional benefit of supplementing the nucleoside uridine with DHA is their combined ability to activate the gene expression of proteins, which, in turn, encourages synapse formation. Some of the brain-related proteins activated by uridine and DHA are: synapsin-1, syntaxin-3 and F-actin (Wurtman et al. 2009).

Therefore, the supplementation of precursor nutrition for synapses appears to be a superior choice compared with supplementing the individual phosphatides. Individual phosphatide supplements (such as phosphatidylcholine, phosphatidylethanolamine and phosphatidylserine) do not activate synaptic genes and usually do not contain DHA, one of the fatty acids preferred by the central nervous system.

Animal products are a rich source of nucleotides and nucleosides, including uridine. Giant oyster mushroom (*Pleurotus gigan-*

teus) are another surprising source of uridine, with experimental evidence supporting their ability to stimulate neurite outgrowth. Other mushrooms, such as Lion's mane, reishi, tiger milk and cordyceps, have all been found to trigger neurite outgrowth and have proven to protect and regenerate neurons (Phan et al. 2015).

The wider benefits of uridine seen in research

Uridine's benefits extend way beyond neurite outgrowth, with positive effects on mitochondrial function, energy, cell membranes and detoxification. As Parkinson's disease patients often suffer from global energy deficits, this research is well worth investigating.

Uridine assists mitochondria to help protect them from calcium overload. Uridine maintains calcium balance by supporting the activity of purine receptors on mitochondrial membranes (Belous et al. 2006). Mitochondrial calcium overload is a major problem in Parkinson's disease patients.

In swim tests, laboratory animals can double their endurance if supplemented with uridine (Mankovskaya et al. 2014).

As an interesting aside, fertility and sperm motility are undermined when seminal fluid is low in uridine. In a similar way to the swim test, improved sperm motility indicates an increase in semen 'swim' energy in the presence of uridine. Fertility also relies on an abundant supply of phospholipids for the rapid synthesis of cell membranes required for growth (Maher et al. 2008). Remember, cell membrane phospholipids are essential to maintain synapse and vesicle integrity in the central nervous system.

Harmful hydrocarbon compounds and metabolites of dopamine can be detoxified by uridine containing UDP-glucuronosyl-transferases (UGTs). UGTs are highly expressed at the blood-brain barrier and in nasal mucosa – two vulnerable areas for xenobiotic entry into the brain (Ouzzine et al. 2014). Xenobiotics are neurotoxic compounds often associated with neurodegeneration.

Uridine is a pyrimidine nucleoside which is dependent on the electron transport chain of mitochondria for its synthesis (Wallace et al. 2010). It is therefore possible that mitochondrial dysfunction may lead to a loss of uridine synthesis, leading to even more mitochondrial defects. Uridine has been shown partially to protect laboratory animals from the mitochondrial damaging effects of the Parkinson's disease-inducing toxin MPTP (1-methyl-4-phenyl-1,2,3,6- tetrahydropyridine) (Wallace et al. 2010).

Other considerations

Vitamin D3 is another nutrient which can stimulate neurite outgrowth. Importantly, vitamin D3 can activate nerve growth factor and protect against misfolded proteins associated with Alzheimer's disease (Littlejohns et al. 2015).

Phospholipid methylation (PLM) is an essential component of phosphatide/phospholipid metabolism. Therefore, supplementation of vitamin B12, B6 and folic acid should be considered alongside uridine, DHA, choline, mushrooms and vitamin D. Furthermore, phospholipid methylation is dependent on dopamine metabolism, as phospholipid methylation requires the involvement of dopamine and D4 dopamine receptors (Sharma et al. 1999); (Zhang et al. 2016).

Exercise is beneficial for neurite outgrowth, and combining exercise with DHA can dramatically amplify the benefits of both. Improved synapse function, axon growth, learning and memory are among the advantages of exercise and dietary DHA (Chytrova et al. 2010).

Bibliography

Abbott, N. J., Rönnbäck, L. and Hansson, E. (2006) 'Astrocyte-endothelial interactions at the blood-brain barrier.', *Nature reviews. Neuroscience*, 7(1), pp. 41–53.

Abou-hamdan, M. *et al.* (2011) 'The Energy Crisis in Parkinson's Disease : A Therapeutic Target', in Rana, P. A. Q. (ed.) *Etiology and Pathophysiology of Parkinson's Disease*. InTech, pp. 273–292.

Adams, J. D., Klaidman, L. K. and Ribeiro, P. (1997) 'Tyrosine hydroxylase: mechanisms of oxygen radical formation.', *Redox report : communications in free radical research*, 3(5–6), pp. 273–9.

Agnati, L. F. *et al.* (2006) 'Allosteric modulation of dopamine D2 receptors by homocysteine.', *Journal of proteome research*. American Chemical Society, 5(11), pp. 3077–83.

Aguzzi, A., Barres, B. a and Bennett, M. L. (2013) 'Microglia: scapegoat, saboteur, or something else?', *Science (New York, N.Y.)*, 339(6116), pp. 156–61.

Ahmad, B. and Lapidus, L. J. (2012) 'Curcumin prevents aggregation in α-synuclein by increasing reconfiguration rate.', *The Journal of biological chemistry*, 287(12), pp. 9193–9. d

Akahoshi, E. *et al.* (2009) 'Effect of dioxins on regulation of tyrosine hydroxylase gene expression by aryl hydrocarbon receptor: a neurotoxicology study.', *Environmental health : a global access science source*, 8, p. 24.

Albanese, A. *et al.* (2013) 'Phenomenology and classification of dystonia: a consensus update.', *Movement disorders : official journal of the Movement Disorder Society*, 28(7), pp. 863–73.

Albers, J. A., Chand, P. and Anch, A. M. (2017) 'Multifactorial sleep disturbance in Parkinson's disease', *Sleep Medicine*. Elsevier, 35, pp. 41–48.

Albert, U. *et al.* (2014) '[Lithium treatment and potential long-term side effects: a systematic review of the literature].', *Rivista di psichiatria*, 49(1), pp. 12–21.

Alfonso-Loeches, S. *et al.* (2010) 'Pivotal role of TLR4 receptors in alcohol-induced neuroinflammation and brain damage.', *The Journal of neuroscience : the official journal of the Society for Neuroscience*, 30(24), pp. 8285–95.

Amadoro, G. *et al.* (2006) 'NMDA receptor mediates tau-induced neurotoxicity by calpain and ERK/MAPK activation.', *Proceedings of the National Academy of Sciences of the United States of America*, 103(8), pp. 2892–7.

Aoyama, K., Watabe, M. and Nakaki, T. (2008) 'Critical Review Regulation of Neuronal Glutathione Synthesis', *J Pharmacol Sci*, 108, pp. 227–238.

Appelqvist, H. *et al.* (2013) 'The lysosome: from waste bag to potential therapeutic target.', *Journal of molecular cell biology*, 5(4), pp. 214–26.

Arevalo, M.-A., Azcoitia, I. and Garcia-Segura, L. M. (2015) 'The neuroprotective actions of oestradiol and oestrogen receptors.', *Nature reviews. Neuroscience*. Nature Publishing Group, a division of Macmillan Publishers Limited. All Rights Reserved., 16(1), pp. 17–29.

Arnoux, J.-B. *et al.* (2013) 'Aromatic L-amino acid decarboxylase deficiency is a cause of long-fasting hypoglycemia.', *The Journal of clinical endocrinology and metabolism*. Endocrine Society Chevy Chase, MD, 98(11), pp. 4279–84.

Atamna, H. *et al.* (2002) 'Heme deficiency may be a factor in the mitochondrial and neuronal decay of aging.', *Proceedings of the National Academy of Sciences of the United States of America*, 99(23), pp. 14807–12.

Atamna, H. (2006) 'Heme binding to Amyloid-beta peptide: mechanistic role in Alzheimer's disease.', *Journal of Alzheimer's disease : JAD*, 10(2–3), pp. 255–66.

Atsmon-Raz, Y. and Miller, Y. (2015) 'Co-Aggregation of Alpha-Synuclein with Amylin(HIAPP) Leads to an Increased Risk in Type ii Diabetes Patients for Developing Parkinson's Disease', *Biophysical Journal*. Biophysical Society, 108(2), p. 524a.

Bánhegyi, G. *et al.* (2003) 'Role of ascorbate in oxidative protein folding.', *BioFactors (Oxford, England)*, 17(1–4), pp. 37–46. Available at: http://www.ncbi.nlm.nih.gov/pubmed/12897427

Barbagallo, M. and Domínguez, L. J. (2013) '[Magnesium, diabetes and metabolic syndrome].', *Cirugía y cirujanos*, 81(5), pp. 365–7. Available at: http://www.ncbi.nlm.nih.gov/pubmed/25125052

Barger, S. W. and Basile, A. S. (2001) 'Activation of microglia by secreted amyloid precursor protein evokes release of glutamate by cystine exchange and attenuates synaptic function.', *Journal of neurochemistry*, 76(3), pp. 846–54. Available at: http://www.ncbi.nlm.nih.gov/pubmed/11158256

Bazan, N. G. (2013) 'The docosanoid neuroprotectin D1 induces homeostatic regulation of neuroinflammation and cell survival.', *Prostaglandins, leukotrienes, and essential fatty acids*, 88(1), pp. 127–9.

Bazinet, R. P. and Layé, S. (2014) 'Polyunsaturated fatty acids and their metabolites in brain function and disease.', *Nature reviews. Neuroscience*, (November).

Bell, E. L. et al. (2007) 'The Qo site of the mitochondrial complex III is required for the transduction of hypoxic signaling via reactive oxygen species production.', *The Journal of cell biology*, 177(6), pp. 1029–36.

Beller, M. et al. (2010) 'Lipid droplets: a dynamic organelle moves into focus.', *FEBS letters*. Federation of European Biochemical Societies, 584(11), pp. 2176–82.

Belous, A. E. et al. (2006) 'Mitochondrial calcium transport is regulated by P2Y1- and P2Y2-like mitochondrial receptors', *Journal of Cellular Biochemistry*. Wiley Subscription Services, Inc., A Wiley Company, 99(4), pp. 1165–1174.

Ben-Shachar, D., Zuk, R. and Glinka, Y. (2002) 'Dopamine Neurotoxicity: Inhibition of Mitochondrial Respiration', *Journal of Neurochemistry*, 64(2), pp. 718–723.

Ben-Zvi, A. P. and Goloubinoff, P. (2001) 'Review: mechanisms of disaggregation and refolding of stable protein aggregates by molecular chaperones.', *Journal of structural biology*, 135(2), pp. 84–93.

Bender, D. A., Earl, C. J. and Lees, A. J. (1979) 'Niacin depletion in Parkinsonian patients treated with L-dopa, benserazide and carbidopa.', *Clinical science (London, England : 1979)*, 56(1), pp. 89–93.

Berman, S. B. and Hastings, T. G. (2001) 'Dopamine Oxidation Alters Mitochondrial Respiration and Induces Permeability Transition in Brain Mitochondria', *Journal of Neurochemistry*, 73(3), pp. 1127–1137.

Bernales, S., Soto, M. and McCullagh, E. (2012) 'Unfolded protein stress in the endoplasmic reticulum and mitochondria: a role in neurodegeneration', *Frontiers in Aging neuroscience*, 4, pp. 1–13.

Bernardo, A. and Minghetti, L. (2006) 'PPAR-gamma agonists as regulators of microglial activation and brain inflammation.', *Current pharmaceutical design*, 12(1), pp. 93–109.

Berry, M. D. and Boulton, A. A. (2013) *Catecholamine Research: From Molecular Insights to Clinical Medicine Volume 53 of Advances in Behavioral Biology*. Edited by T. Nagatsu et al. Springer Science & Business Media.

Bhattacharyya, R., Barren, C. and Kovacs, D. M. (2013) 'Palmitoylation of amyloid precursor protein regulates amyloidogenic processing in lipid rafts.', *The Journal of neuroscience : the official journal of the Society for Neuroscience*, 33(27), pp. 11169–83.

Bisaglia, M. *et al.* (2013) 'Dysfunction of dopamine homeostasis: clues in the hunt for novel Parkinson's disease therapies.', *FASEB journal : official publication of the Federation of American Societies for Experimental Biology*, 27(6), pp. 2101–10.

Björkhem, I. *et al.* (2013) 'Oxysterols and Parkinson's disease: evidence that levels of 24S-hydroxycholesterol in cerebrospinal fluid correlates with the duration of the disease.', *Neuroscience letters*, 555, pp. 102–5. doi: 10.1016/j.neulet.2013.09.003.

Block, M. L., Zecca, L. and Hong, J.-S. (2007) 'Microglia-mediated neurotoxicity: uncovering the molecular mechanisms.', *Nature reviews. Neuroscience*, 8(1), pp. 57–69.

Boslem, E. *et al.* (2013) 'Alteration of endoplasmic reticulum lipid rafts contributes to lipotoxicity in pancreatic β-cells.', *The Journal of biological chemistry*, 288(37), pp. 26569–82.

Bourassa, M. W. and Miller, L. M. (2012) 'Metal imaging in neurodegenerative diseases.', *Metallomics : integrated biometal science*, 4(8), pp. 721–38.

Bozic, I. *et al.* (2015) 'Benfotiamine attenuates inflammatory response in LPS stimulated BV-2 microglia.', *PloS one*, 10(2), p. e0118372.

Braidy, N. *et al.* (2010) 'Neuroprotective effects of naturally occurring polyphenols on quinolinic acid-induced excitotoxicity in human neurons.', *The FEBS journal*, 277(2), pp. 368–82.

Branco, A. F. *et al.* (2016) 'Ketogenic diets: From cancer to mitochondrial diseases and beyond', *European Journal of Clinical Investigation*, pp. 285–298.

Brenna, J. T. *et al.* (2009) 'alpha-Linolenic acid supplementation and conversion to n-3 long-chain polyunsaturated fatty acids in humans.', *Prostaglandins, leukotrienes, and essential fatty acids*, 80(2–3), pp. 85–91.

Burg, J. S. and Espenshade, P. J. (2011) 'Regulation of HMG-CoA reductase in mammals and yeast.', *Progress in lipid research*, 50(4), pp. 403–10.

Burke, W. J. (2003) '3,4-dihydroxyphenylacetaldehyde: a potential target for neuroprotective therapy in Parkinson's disease.', *Current drug targets. CNS and neurological disorders*, 2(2), pp. 143–8.

Cabezas, R. et al. (2014) 'Astrocytic modulation of blood brain barrier: perspectives on Parkinson's disease.', *Frontiers in cellular neuroscience*. Frontiers, 8, p. 211.

Calderón-Montaño, J. M. et al. (2011) 'A review on the dietary flavonoid kaempferol.', *Mini reviews in medicinal chemistry*, 11(4), pp. 298–344.

Calì, T. et al. (2012) 'α-Synuclein controls mitochondrial calcium homeostasis by enhancing endoplasmic reticulum-mitochondria interactions.', *The Journal of biological chemistry*, 287(22), pp. 17914–29.

Cansev, M. et al. (2008) 'Restorative effects of uridine plus docosahexaenoic acid in a rat model of Parkinson's disease', *Neuroscience Research*, 62(3), pp. 206–209.

Carey, A. N. et al. (2013) 'Stilbenes and anthocyanins reduce stress signaling in BV-2 mouse microglia.', *Journal of agricultural and food chemistry*, 61(25), pp. 5979–86.

Carmona-Ramírez, I. et al. (2012) 'Curcumin restores Nrf2 levels and prevents quinolinic acid-induced neurotoxicity.', *The Journal of nutritional biochemistry*, null(null).

Carradori, S. et al. (2014) 'Selective MAO-B inhibitors: a lesson from natural products.', *Molecular diversity*, 18(1), pp. 219–43.

Caruana, M. et al. (2011) 'Inhibition and disaggregation of α-synuclein oligomers by natural polyphenolic compounds.', *FEBS letters*. Federation of European Biochemical Societies, 585(8), pp. 1113–20.

Cavalieri, E. L. et al. (2002) 'Catechol ortho-quinones: the electrophilic compounds that form depurinating DNA adducts and could initiate cancer and other diseases.', *Carcinogenesis*, 23(6), pp. 1071–7.

Chankova, S. et al. (2013) 'Heat shock protein HSP70B as a marker for genotype resistance to environmental stress in Chlorella species from contrasting habitats.', *Gene*, 516(1), pp. 184–9. d

Charan, R. A. *et al.* (2014) 'Inhibition of apoptotic Bax translocation to the mitochondria is a central function of parkin.', *Cell death & disease*. Macmillan Publishers Limited, 5, p. e1313.

Charlton, C. G. and Mack, J. (1994) 'Substantia nigra degeneration and tyrosine hydroxylase depletion caused by excess S-adenosylmethionine in the rat brain. Support for an excess methylation hypothesis for parkinsonism.', *Molecular neurobiology*, 9(1–3), pp. 149–61.

Chaudhary, S. and Parvez, S. (2012) 'An in vitro approach to assess the neurotoxicity of valproic acid-induced oxidative stress in cerebellum and cerebral cortex of young rats.', *Neuroscience*, 225, pp. 258–68.

Chen, L. *et al.* (2008) 'Manufactured aluminum oxide nanoparticles decrease expression of tight junction proteins in brain vasculature.', *Journal of neuroimmune pharmacology : the official journal of the Society on NeuroImmune Pharmacology*, 3(4), pp. 286–95.

Chen, X., Ghribi, O. and Geiger, J. D. (2010) 'Caffeine protects against disruptions of the blood-brain barrier in animal models of Alzheimer's and Parkinson's diseases.', *Journal of Alzheimer's disease : JAD*, 20 Suppl 1, pp. S127-41.

Chinta, S. J. and Andersen, J. K. (2011) 'Nitrosylation and nitration of mitochondrial complex I in Parkinson's disease.', *Free radical research*. Informa Healthcare London, 45(1), pp. 53–8.

Choi, D. K., Koppula, S. and Suk, K. (2011) 'Inhibitors of microglial neurotoxicity: focus on natural products.', *Molecules (Basel, Switzerland)*, 16(2), pp. 1021–43.

Choi, S. Y. *et al.* (1999) 'Hydrogen peroxide-mediated Cu,Zn-superoxide dismutase fragmentation: protection by carnosine, homocarnosine and anserine', *Biochimica et Biophysica Acta (BBA) - General Subjects*, 1472(3), pp. 651–657.

Chu, Y. *et al.* (2009) 'Alterations in lysosomal and proteasomal markers in Parkinson's disease: relationship to alpha-synuclein inclusions.', *Neurobiology of disease*, 35(3), pp. 385–98.

Chytrova, G., Ying, Z. and Gomez-Pinilla, F. (2010) 'Exercise contributes to the effects of DHA dietary supplementation by acting on membrane-related synaptic systems', *Brain Research*, 1341, pp. 32–40.

Clementi, F. M. (2006) *Interaction between dopamine and histamine in the basal ganglia*. Karolinska Institutet.

Daidone, F. *et al.* (2012) 'Identification by virtual screening and in vitro testing of human DOPA decarboxylase inhibitors.', *PloS one*. Public Library of Science, 7(2), p. e31610. d

Dall'Armi, C., Devereaux, K. A. and Di Paolo, G. (2013) 'The role of lipids in the control of autophagy.', *Current biology : CB*, 23(1), pp. R33-45.

Dauer, W. and Przedborski, S. (2003) 'Parkinson ' s Disease : Mechanisms and Models', *Neuron*, 39(6), pp. 889–909.

Davenward, S. *et al.* (2013) 'Silicon-rich mineral water as a non-invasive test of the "aluminum hypothesis" in Alzheimer's disease.', *Journal of Alzheimer's disease : JAD*, 33(2), pp. 423–30.

Davis, J. M. *et al.* (2009) 'Quercetin increases brain and muscle mitochondrial biogenesis and exercise tolerance.', *American journal of physiology. Regulatory, integrative and comparative physiology*, 296(4), pp. R1071-7.

Dedkova, E. N. and Blatter, L. A. (2014) 'Role of β-hydroxybutyrate, its polymer poly-β-hydroxybutyrate and inorganic polyphosphate in mammalian health and disease', *Frontiers in Physiology*. Frontiers, 5 JUL, p. 260.

Dehay, B. *et al.* (2010) 'Pathogenic lysosomal depletion in Parkinson's disease.', *The Journal of neuroscience : the official journal of the Society for Neuroscience*, 30(37), pp. 12535–44.

Devi, L. *et al.* (2008) 'Mitochondrial import and accumulation of alpha-synuclein impair complex I in human dopaminergic neuronal cultures and Parkinson disease brain.', *The Journal of biological chemistry*, 283(14), pp. 9089–100.

Dhatariya, K. and Savage, M. (2013) *The Management of Diabetic ketoacidosis in adults*, Joint British Diabetes Societies Inpatient care group.

Diepenbroek, M. *et al.* (2014) 'Overexpression of the calpain-specific inhibitor calpastatin reduces human alpha-Synuclein processing, aggregation and synaptic impairment in [A30P]αSyn transgenic mice.', *Human molecular genetics*. Oxford University Press, 23(15), pp. 3975–89.

Dinkova-Kostova, A. T. and Talalay, P. (2010) 'NAD(P)H:quinone acceptor oxidoreductase 1 (NQO1), a multifunctional antioxidant enzyme and exceptionally versatile cytoprotector.', *Archives of biochemistry and biophysics*, 501(1), pp. 116–23.

Dolhun, A. (2015) 'Levodopa 2.0: New Strategies to Even Out the Peaks and Valleys', *Practical Neurology*, 06, pp. 26–29.

Dowd, P. and Zheng, Z. B. (1995) 'On the mechanism of the anticlotting action of vitamin E quinone.', *Proceedings of the National Academy of Sciences of the United States of America*, 92(18), pp. 8171–5.

Drake, T. M. (2015) 'Unfolding the Promise of Translational Targeting in Neurodegenerative Disease.', *Neuromolecular medicine*.

Dreiseitel, A. *et al.* (2009) 'Berry anthocyanins and their aglycons inhibit monoamine oxidases A and B.', *Pharmacological research : the official journal of the Italian Pharmacological Society*, 59(5), pp. 306–11.

Du, J. *et al.* (2009) 'PPARγ transcriptionally regulates the expression of insulin-degrading enzyme in primary neurons', *Biochemical and Biophysical Research Communications*, 383(4), pp. 485–490.

Eisenhofer, G., Kopin, I. and Goldstein, D. (2004) 'Catecholamine metabolism: a contemporary view with implications for physiology and medicine', *Pharmacological reviews*, 56(3), pp. 331–349.

Exley, C. (2014) 'Why industry propaganda and political interference cannot disguise the inevitable role played by human exposure to aluminum in neurodegenerative diseases, including Alzheimer's disease.', *Frontiers in neurology*, 5, p. 212.

Fabelo, N. *et al.* (2011) 'Severe alterations in lipid composition of frontal cortex lipid rafts from Parkinson's disease and incidental Parkinson's disease.', *Molecular medicine (Cambridge, Mass.)*, 17(9–10), pp. 1107–18.

Fagone, P. and Jackowski, S. (2009) 'Membrane phospholipid synthesis and endoplasmic reticulum function.', *Journal of lipid research*, 50 Suppl, pp. S311-6.

Fahn, S. (2000) 'The spectrum of levodopa-induced dyskinesias.', *Annals of neurology*, 47(4 Suppl 1), pp. S2-9; discussion S9-11. Available at: http://europepmc.org/abstract/med/10762127

Farokhi, M. *et al.* (2014) 'Role of histamine and diamine oxidase enzyme in Multiple Sclerosis', *Multiple Sclerosis and Related Disorders*. Elsevier, 3(6), p. 746.

Farooqui, A. A. (2006) 'Inhibitors of Brain Phospholipase A2 Activity: Their Neuropharmacological Effects and Therapeutic Importance for the Treatment of Neurologic Disorders', *Pharmacological Reviews*. American Society for Pharmacology and Experimental Therapeutics, 58(3), pp. 591–620.

Fasano, A. (2011) 'Zonulin and its regulation of intestinal barrier function: the biological door to inflammation, autoimmunity, and cancer.', *Physiological reviews*, 91(1), pp. 151–75.

Faustino, J. V *et al.* (2011) 'Microglial cells contribute to endogenous brain defenses after acute neonatal focal stroke.', *The Journal of neuroscience : the official journal of the Society for Neuroscience*, 31(36), pp. 12992–3001.

Ferrari-Toninelli, G. *et al.* (2008) 'Dopamine receptor agonists for protection and repair in Parkinson's disease.', *Current topics in medicinal chemistry*, 8(12), pp. 1089–99.

Filipov, N. M. and Dodd, C. a (2012) 'Role of glial cells in manganese neurotoxicity.', *Journal of applied toxicology : JAT*, 32(5), pp. 310–7.

Forsyth, C. B. *et al.* (2011) 'Increased intestinal permeability correlates with sigmoid mucosa alpha-synuclein staining and endotoxin exposure markers in early Parkinson's disease.', *PloS one*, 6(12), p. e28032.

Foulds, P. G. *et al.* (2013) 'A longitudinal study on α-synuclein in blood plasma as a biomarker for Parkinson's disease.', *Scientific reports*, 3(2540), pp. 1–6.

De Franceschi, G. *et al.* (2011) 'Structural and morphological characterization of aggregated species of α-synuclein induced by docosahexaenoic acid.', *The Journal of biological chemistry*, 286(25), pp. 22262–74.

Fröhlich, M. *et al.* (2014) 'S-palmitoylation represents a novel mechanism regulating the mitochondrial targeting of BAX and initiation of apoptosis.', *Cell death & disease*. Macmillan Publishers Limited, 5, p. e1057.

Fujiyama-Fujiwara, Y., Umeda, R. and Igarashi, O. (1992) 'Effects of sesamin and curcumin on delta 5-desaturation and chain elongation of polyunsaturated fatty acid metabolism in primary cultured rat hepatocytes.', *Journal of nutritional science and vitaminology*, 38(4), pp. 353–63. Av ailable at: http://www.ncbi.nlm.nih.gov/pubmed/1291640

Gaikwad, N. W. *et al.* (2011) 'Imbalanced estrogen metabolism in the brain: possible relevance to the etiology of Parkinson's disease.', *Biomarkers : biochemical indicators of exposure, response, and susceptibility to chemicals*, 16(5), pp. 434–44.

Gao, X. (2012) 'Prospective Study of Statin Use and Risk of Parkinson Disease', *Archives of Neurology*. American Medical Association, 69(3), p. 380.

García, O. P., Long, K. Z. and Rosado, J. L. (2009) 'Impact of micronutrient deficiencies on obesity.', *Nutrition reviews*. The Oxford University Press, 67(10), pp. 559-72.

Gasche, Y. *et al.* (2001) 'Matrix metalloproteinase inhibition prevents oxidative stress-associated blood-brain barrier disruption after transient focal cerebral ischemia.', *Journal of cerebral blood flow and metabolism : official journal of the International Society of Cerebral Blood Flow and Metabolism*, 21(12), pp. 1393-400.

Gasior, M., Rogawski, M. A. and Hartman, A. L. (2006) 'Neuroprotective and disease-modifying effects of the ketogenic diet.', *Behavioural pharmacology*, 17(5-6), pp. 431-9.

Gélinas, S. and Martinoli, M.-G. (2002) 'Neuroprotective effect of estradiol and phytoestrogens on MPP+-induced cytotoxicity in neuronal PC12 cells.', *Journal of neuroscience research*, 70(1), pp. 90-6.

Geng, X. *et al.* (2011) 'α-Synuclein binds the K(ATP) channel at insulin-secretory granules and inhibits insulin secretion.', *American journal of physiology. Endocrinology and metabolism*, 300(2), pp. E276-86.

George, K. S. and Wu, S. (2012) 'Lipid raft: A floating island of death or survival.', *Toxicology and applied pharmacology*, 259(3), pp. 311-9.

Gerster, H. (1998) 'Can adults adequately convert alpha-linolenic acid (18:3n-3) to eicosapentaenoic acid (20:5n-3) and docosahexaenoic acid (22:6n-3)?', *International journal for vitamin and nutrition research. Internationale Zeitschrift für Vitamin- und Ernährungsforschung. Journal international de vitaminologie et de nutrition*, 68(3), pp. 159-73.

Gibrat, C. *et al.* (2009) 'Differences between subacute and chronic MPTP mice models: investigation of dopaminergic neuronal degeneration and alpha-synuclein inclusions.', *Journal of neurochemistry*, 109(5), pp. 1469-82.

Goldstein, D. S. *et al.* (2013) 'Determinants of buildup of the toxic dopamine metabolite DOPAL in Parkinson's disease.', *Journal of neurochemistry*, 126(5), pp. 591-603.

Gomes, M. B. and Negrato, C. A. (2014) 'Alpha-lipoic acid as a pleiotropic compound with potential therapeutic use in diabetes and other chronic diseases.', *Diabetology & metabolic syndrome*, 6(1), p. 80.

Goodman, J. E. (2001) 'COMT genotype, micronutrients in the folate metabolic pathway and breast cancer risk', *Carcinogenesis*, 22(10), pp. 1661–1665.

Grasso, G. *et al.* (2011) 'Copper(I) and copper(II) inhibit Aβ peptides proteolysis by insulin-degrading enzyme differently: implications for metallostasis alteration in Alzheimer's disease.', *Chemistry (Weinheim an der Bergstrasse, Germany)*, 17(9), pp. 2752–62.

Gruber, F. *et al.* (2015) 'Nrf2 deficiency causes lipid oxidation, inflammation, and matrix-protease expression in DHA-supplemented and UVA-irradiated skin fibroblasts.', *Free radical biology & medicine*, 88(Pt B), pp. 439–51.

Grygiel-Górniak, B. (2014) 'Peroxisome proliferator-activated receptors and their ligands: nutritional and clinical implications--a review.', *Nutrition journal*, 13, p. 17.

Guardia-Laguarta, C. *et al.* (2014) 'α-Synuclein is localized to mitochondria-associated ER membranes.', *The Journal of neuroscience : the official journal of the Society for Neuroscience*, 34(1), pp. 249–59.

Guardia-Laguarta, C. *et al.* (2015) 'Novel subcellular localization for α-synuclein: possible functional consequences.', *Frontiers in neuroanatomy*, 9, p. 17.

Gupta, V. *et al.* (2013) 'Salicylic acid induces mitochondrial injury by inhibiting ferrochelatase heme biosynthesis activity.', *Molecular pharmacology*, 84(6), pp. 824–33.

Habashi, S., Sabouni, F. and Moghimi, A. (2012) 'Reduction of NO production in LPS-stimulated primary rat microglial cells by Bromelain', *profdoc.um.ac.ir*, 3(2), pp. 57–65.

Habib, C. N. *et al.* (2015) 'Leptin influences estrogen metabolism and accelerates prostate cell proliferation.', *Life sciences*, 121, pp. 10–5.

Han, S. *et al.* (2012) 'Resveratrol upregulated heat shock proteins and extended the survival of G93A-SOD1 mice.', *Brain research*, 1483, pp. 112–7.

Haorah, J. *et al.* (2005) 'Alcohol-induced oxidative stress in brain endothelial cells causes blood-brain barrier dysfunction.', *Journal of leukocyte biology*, 78(6), pp. 1223–32.

Hayden, E. Y. *et al.* (2015) 'Heme Stabilization of α-Synuclein Oligomers during Amyloid Fibril Formation.', *Biochemistry*, 54(30), pp. 4599–610.

He, H.-J. *et al.* (2012) 'Curcumin attenuates Nrf2 signaling defect, oxidative stress in muscle and glucose intolerance in high fat diet-fed mice.', *World journal of diabetes*, 3(5), pp. 94–104.

Hellmann-Regen, J. *et al.* (2013) 'Accelerated degradation of retinoic acid by activated microglia', *Journal of Neuroimmunology*, 256(1–2), pp. 1–6.

Hicks, D. A., Nalivaeva, N. N. and Turner, A. J. (2012) 'Lipid rafts and Alzheimer's disease: protein-lipid interactions and perturbation of signaling.', *Frontiers in physiology*, 3, p. 189.

Hinz, M., Stein, A. and Cole, T. (2014a) 'Parkinson's disease: carbidopa, nausea, and dyskinesia.', *Clinical pharmacology : advances and applications*, 6, pp. 189–94.

Hinz, M., Stein, A. and Cole, T. (2014b) 'The Parkinson's disease death rate: carbidopa and vitamin B6.', *Clinical pharmacology : advances and applications*, 6, pp. 161–9.

Hirrlinger, J. *et al.* (2000) 'Microglial cells in culture express a prominent glutathione system for the defense against reactive oxygen species.', *Developmental neuroscience*, 22(5–6), pp. 384–92.

Holemans, T. *et al.* (2015) 'A lipid switch unlocks Parkinson's disease-associated ATP13A2.', *Proceedings of the National Academy of Sciences of the United States of America*, 112(29), pp. 9040–5.

Holroyd, S. and Smith, D. (1995) 'Disabling Parkinsonism Due to Lithium: A Case Report', *Journal of Geriatric Psychiatry and Neurology*, 8(2), pp. 118–119.

Hood, M. I. and Skaar, E. P. (2012) 'Nutritional immunity: transition metals at the pathogen-host interface.', *Nature reviews. Microbiology*, 10(8), pp. 525–37.

Hsiao, G. *et al.* (2004) 'A potent antioxidant, lycopene, affords neuroprotection against microglia activation and focal cerebral ischemia in rats', *in vivo*, 356, pp. 351–356.

Hussain, G. *et al.* (2013) 'Fatting the brain: a brief of recent research.', *Frontiers in cellular neuroscience*, 7, p. 144.

Hwang, Y. P. and Jeong, H. G. (2010) 'Ginsenoside Rb1 protects against 6-hydroxydopamine-induced oxidative stress by increasing heme oxygenase-1 expression through an estrogen receptor-related PI3K/Akt/Nrf2-dependent pathway in human dopaminergic cells.', *Toxicology and applied pharmacology*, 242(1), pp. 18–28.

Imam, S. Z. et al. (2013) 'Neuroprotective efficacy of a new brain-penetrating C-Abl inhibitor in a murine Parkinson's disease model.', *PloS one*. Public Library of Science, 8(5), p. e65129.

Innamorato, N. G. et al. (2008) 'The Transcription Factor Nrf2 Is a Therapeutic Target against Brain Inflammation', *The Journal of Immunology*. American Association of Immunologists, 181(1), pp. 680–689.

Ito, T., Schaffer, S. W. and Azuma, J. (2012) 'The potential usefulness of taurine on diabetes mellitus and its complications.', *Amino acids*, 42(5), pp. 1529–39.

Jackson, K. et al. (2013) 'Amylin deposition in the brain: A second amyloid in Alzheimer disease?', *Annals of neurology*, 74(4), pp. 517–26.

Jana, S. et al. (2011) 'Mitochondrial dysfunction mediated by quinone oxidation products of dopamine: Implications in dopamine cytotoxicity and pathogenesis of Parkinson's disease.', *Biochimica et biophysica acta*, 1812(6), pp. 663–73.

Janik, M. E., Bełkot, K. and Przybyło, M. (2014) 'Review Is oestrogen an important player in melanoma progression?', *Współczesna Onkologia*, 5(5), pp. 302–306.

Jensen, S. K. and Yong, V. W. (2014) 'Microglial modulation as a mechanism behind the promotion of central nervous system well-being by physical exercise', *Clinical and Experimental Neuroimmunology*, 5(2), pp. 188–201.

Jiang, T. et al. (2015) 'P2X7 receptor is critical in α-synuclein-mediated microglial NADPH oxidase activation.', *Neurobiology of aging*. Elsevier, 36(7), pp. 2304–18.

Jo, Y. and Debose-Boyd, R. A. (2010) 'Control of cholesterol synthesis through regulated ER-associated degradation of HMG CoA reductase.', *Critical reviews in biochemistry and molecular biology*, 45(3), pp. 185–98.

Johansen, J. L. et al. (2010) 'HIF prolyl hydroxylase inhibition increases cell viability and potentiates dopamine release in dopaminergic cells.', *Journal of neurochemistry*, 115(1), pp. 209–19.

Johnson, C. J. et al. (2011) 'Meat and bone meal and mineral feed additives may increase the risk of oral prion disease transmission.', *Journal of toxicology and environmental health. Part A*. Taylor & Francis Group, 74(2–4), pp. 161–6.

Johnson, R. J. et al. (2005) 'Uric acid, evolution and primitive cultures', *Seminars in Nephrology*, 25(1), pp. 3–8.

Jong, C. J., Azuma, J. and Schaffer, S. (2012) 'Mechanism underlying the antioxidant activity of taurine: prevention of mitochondrial oxidant production.', *Amino acids*, 42(6), pp. 2223–32.

Kang, J. H. and Kim, K. S. (2003) 'Enhanced oligomerization of the alpha-synuclein mutant by the Cu,Zn-superoxide dismutase and hydrogen peroxide system.', *Molecules and cells*, 15(1), pp. 87–93.

Kapitein, L. C. and Hoogenraad, C. C. (2015) 'Building the Neuronal Microtubule Cytoskeleton', *Neuron*. Elsevier, 87(3), pp. 492–506.

Kapitein, L. C. and Hoogenraad, C. C. (2015) 'Building the Neuronal Microtubule Cytoskeleton', *Neuron*, pp. 492–506.

Kareus, S. A. *et al.* (2012) 'Shared predispositions of parkinsonism and cancer: a population-based pedigree-linked study.', *Archives of neurology*, 69(12), pp. 1572–7.

Karuppagounder, S. S. *et al.* (2014) 'The c-Abl inhibitor, nilotinib, protects dopaminergic neurons in a preclinical animal model of Parkinson's disease.', *Scientific reports*, 4, p. 4874.

Katzenschlager, R. *et al.* (2004) 'Mucuna pruriens in Parkinson's disease: a double blind clinical and pharmacological study.', *Journal of neurology, neurosurgery, and psychiatry*, 75(12), pp. 1672–7.

Kauppinen, T. M. *et al.* (2008) 'Zinc triggers microglial activation.', *The Journal of neuroscience : the official journal of the Society for Neuroscience*, 28(22), pp. 5827–35.

Kavyaa, R. K. and Dikshit, M. (2005) 'Role of Nitric Oxide/Nitric Oxide Synthase in Parkinson's Disease', *Annals of Neurosciences*, 12(2), pp. 1–5.

Keen, C. L. *et al.* (1980) 'Regulation of superoxide dismutase activity by dietary manganese . Regulation of Superoxide', *Journal of Nutrition*, 110(4), pp. 795–804.

Keeney, P. M. *et al.* (2006) 'Parkinson's disease brain mitochondrial complex I has oxidatively damaged subunits and is functionally impaired and misassembled.', *The Journal of neuroscience : the official journal of the Society for Neuroscience*, 26(19), pp. 5256–64.

Khwaja, G. and Ranjan, R. (2010) 'Valproate-induced reversible "parkinsonism plus" syndrome', *Journal, Indian Academy of Clinical Medicine*, 11(3), pp. 235–238.

Kim, C. S. and Ross, I. A. (2014) 'Regulatory Role of Free Fatty Acids (FFAs)— Palmitoylation and Myristoylation', *Food and Nutrition Sciences*, 4(9A), pp. 202–211.

Kim, D. Y. *et al.* (2015) 'Ketone bodies mediate antiseizure effects through mitochondrial permeability transition', *Annals of Neurology*, 78(1), pp. 77–87.

Kim, H.-J. *et al.* (2008) 'Liver X receptor beta (LXRbeta): a link between beta-sitosterol and amyotrophic lateral sclerosis-Parkinson's dementia.', *Proceedings of the National Academy of Sciences of the United States of America*, 105(6), pp. 2094–9.

Kim, H. W. *et al.* (2014) '3,3'-Diindolylmethane inhibits lipopolysaccharide-induced microglial hyperactivation and attenuates brain inflammation.', *Toxicological sciences : an official journal of the Society of Toxicology*, 137(1), pp. 158–67.

Kim, I.-S. *et al.* (2011) 'Protective effect of Chrysanthemum indicum Linne against 1-methyl-4-phenylpridinium ion and lipopolysaccharide-induced cytotoxicity in cellular model of Parkinson's disease.', *Food and chemical toxicology : an international journal published for the British Industrial Biological Research Association*, 49(4), pp. 963–73.

Kim, K. S. *et al.* (2002) 'The ceruloplasmin and hydrogen peroxide system induces α-synuclein aggregation in vitro', *Biochimie*, 84(7), pp. 625–631.

Kim, M. *et al.* (2014) 'Berberine prevents nigrostriatal dopaminergic neuronal loss and suppresses hippocampal apoptosis in mice with Parkinson's disease.', *International journal of molecular medicine*, 33(4), pp. 870–8.

Kim, S. T. *et al.* (2005) 'Immobilization stress causes increases in tetrahydrobiopterin, dopamine, and neuromelanin and oxidative damage in the nigrostriatal system.', *Journal of neurochemistry*, 95(1), pp. 89–98.

Klein, P., Tyrlikova, I. and Mathews, G. C. (2014) 'Dietary treatment in adults with refractory epilepsy: A review.', *Neurology*, 83(21), pp. 1978–1985.

Kubo, S. *et al.* (2005) 'A combinatorial code for the interaction of alpha-synuclein with membranes.', *The Journal of biological chemistry*, 280(36), pp. 31664–72.

Kubo, S., Hatano, T. and Hattori, N. (2015) 'Lipid rafts involvement in the pathogenesis of Parkinson's disease.', *Frontiers in bioscience (Landmark edition)*, 20, pp. 263–79.

Kuhn, D. M. *et al.* (1999) 'Tyrosine Hydroxylase Is Inactivated by Catechol-Quinones and Converted to a Redox-Cycling Quinoprotein : Possible Relevance to Parkinson ' s Disease', *Journal of Neurochemistry*, 73(3), pp. 1309–1317.

Kumar, P., Kale, R. and Baquer, N. (2015) 'Mechanisms for the Protective Effects of 17-beta-estradiol: Relevance to Depressive Symptoms in Parkinson's Disease.', *European Psychiatry*, 30, p. 601.

Kupfer, L., Hinrichs, W. and Groschup, M. H. (2009) 'Prion protein misfolding.', *Current molecular medicine*, 9(7), pp. 826–35.

Lai, P.-L. *et al.* (2013) 'Neurotrophic Properties of the Lion's Mane Medicinal Mushroom, Hericium erinaceus (Higher Basidiomycetes) from Malaysia', *International Journal of Medicinal Mushrooms*. Begel House Inc., 15(6), pp. 539–554.

de Lau, L. M. L. *et al.* (2005) 'Dietary fatty acids and the risk of Parkinson disease: the Rotterdam study.', *Neurology*, 64(12), pp. 2040–5.

Lawrence, M. *et al.* (2015) 'Oestrogen receptor α promotes prostate cancer progression through dual actions in both epithelia and stroma', *Endocrine Abstracts*. BioScientifica.

Lee, H.-J. *et al.* (2010) 'Brain arachidonic acid cascade enzymes are upregulated in a rat model of unilateral Parkinson disease.', *Neurochemical research*, 35(4), pp. 613–9.

Lee, K.-W. *et al.* (2011) 'Enhanced phosphatase activity attenuates α-synucleinopathy in a mouse model.', *The Journal of neuroscience : the official journal of the Society for Neuroscience*, 31(19), pp. 6963–71.

Lee, K.-W. *et al.* (2013) 'Neuroprotective and anti-inflammatory properties of a coffee component in the MPTP model of Parkinson's disease.', *Neurotherapeutics : the journal of the American Society for Experimental NeuroTherapeutics*, 10(1), pp. 143–53.

Lee, S.-K. *et al.* (2014) 'Hyperforin attenuates microglia activation and inhibits p65-Ser276 NFκB phosphorylation in the rat piriform cortex following status epilepticus.', *Neuroscience research*, 85, pp. 39–50.

Lee, Y.-H. *et al.* (2015) 'Aryl hydrocarbon receptor mediates both proinflammatory and anti-inflammatory effects in lipopolysaccharide-activated microglia.', *Glia*, 63(7), pp. 1138–54.

Lema Tomé, C. M. *et al.* (2012) 'Inflammation and α-Synuclein's Prion-like Behavior in Parkinson's Disease-Is There a Link?', *Molecular neurobiology*.

Lemaire-Ewing, S. *et al.* (2010) 'Vitamin E transport, membrane incorporation and cell metabolism: Is α-tocopherol in lipid rafts an oar in the lifeboat?', *Molecular Nutrition & Food Research*, 54(5), pp. 631–640.

Leranth, C. *et al.* (2000) 'Estrogen is essential for maintaining nigrostriatal dopamine neurons in primates: implications for Parkinson's disease and memory.', *The Journal of neuroscience : the official journal of the Society for Neuroscience*, 20(23), pp. 8604–9.

Leunbach, T. L. *et al.* (2014) 'Acute favism: methemoglobinemia may cause cyanosis and low pulse oximetry readings.', *Pediatric hematology and oncology*. Informa Healthcare New York, 31(1), pp. 104–6.

Lewis, P. A. and Cookson, M. R. (2012) 'Gene expression in the Parkinson's disease brain.', *Brain research bulletin*, 88(4), pp. 302–12.

Li, Q. *et al.* (2005) 'Docosahexaenoic acid changes lipid composition and interleukin-2 receptor signaling in membrane rafts.', *Journal of lipid research*, 46(9), pp. 1904–13.

Li, X. *et al.* (2001) 'Mitochondrial uptake and recycling of ascorbic acid.', *Archives of biochemistry and biophysics*, 387(1), pp. 143–53.

Li, Y. *et al.* (2001) 'Vitamin E suppression of microglial activation is neuroprotective', *Journal of Neuroscience Research*. John Wiley & Sons, Inc., 66(2), pp. 163–170.

Lindholm, D., Wootz, H. and Korhonen, L. (2006) 'ER stress and neurodegenerative diseases.', *Cell death and differentiation*, 13(3), pp. 385–92.

Di Lisa, F., Menabo, R. and Carpi, A. (2014) 'P429 * The activity of monoamine oxidases is tightly related to mitochondrial membrane fluidity altered by aging, obesity and oxidative stress', *Cardiovascular Research*, 103(suppl 1), pp. S79–S79.

Littlejohns, T. J. *et al.* (2015) 'Vitamin D and Dementia', *J Prev Alz Dis*.

Liu, B. (2006) 'Modulation of Microglial Pro-in fl ammatory and Neurotoxic Activity for the Treatment of Parkinson ' s Disease', *AAPS Journal*, 8(3), pp. 606–621.

Liu, M.-C. *et al.* (2012) 'Involvement of microglia activation in the lead induced long-term potentiation impairment.', *PloS one*, 7(8), p. e43924.

Liu, X. et al. (2008) 'DHA Hydroperoxides as a Potential Inducer of Neuronal Cell Death: a Mitochondrial Dysfunction-Mediated Pathway', *Journal of Clinical Biochemistry and Nutrition*, 43(1), pp. 26–33.

Long, T. C. et al. (2006) 'Titanium Dioxide (P25) Produces Reactive Oxygen Species in Immortalized Brain Microglia (BV2): Implications for Nanoparticle Neurotoxicity †', *Environmental Science & Technology*. American Chemical Society, 40(14), pp. 4346–4352.

Lotharius, J. and Brundin, P. (2002) 'Impaired dopamine storage resulting from a-synuclein mutations may contribute to the pathogenesis of Parkinson ' s disease', 11(20), pp. 2395–2407.

Lou, J.-S. et al. (2001) 'Exacerbated physical fatigue and mental fatigue in Parkinson's disease', *Movement Disorders*, 16(2), pp. 190–196.

Ludvik, B. et al. (1997) 'Amylin: history and overview.', *Diabetic medicine : a journal of the British Diabetic Association*, 14 Suppl 2, pp. S9-13.

Luk, K. C. and Lee, V. M.-Y. (2014) 'Modeling Lewy pathology propagation in Parkinson's disease.', *Parkinsonism & related disorders*, 20 Suppl 1, pp. S85-7.

Ma, D. W. L. et al. (2004) 'n-3 PUFA and membrane microdomains: a new frontier in bioactive lipid research.', *The Journal of nutritional biochemistry*, 15(11), pp. 700–6.

Macht, M. and Ellgring, H. (1999) 'Behavioral analysis of the freezing phenomenon in Parkinson's disease: a case study', *Journal of Behavior Therapy and Experimental Psychiatry*, 30(3), pp. 241–247.

Maden, M. (2007) 'Retinoic acid in the development, regeneration and maintenance of the nervous system', *Nature reviews. Neuroscience*. Nature Publishing Group, 8(10), pp. 755–765.

Madore, C. et al. (2014) 'Nutritional n-3 PUFAs deficiency during perinatal periods alters brain innate immune system and neuronal plasticity-associated genes.', *Brain, behavior, and immunity*, 41, pp. 22–31.

Maher, A. D. et al. (2008) 'Seminal oligouridinosis: Low uridine secretion as a biomarker for infertility in spinal neurotrauma', *Clinical Chemistry*, 54(12), pp. 2063–2066.

Mahul-Mellier, A.-L. et al. (2014) 'c-Abl phosphorylates α-synuclein and regulates its degradation: implication for α-synuclein clearance and contribution to the pathogenesis of Parkinson's disease.', *Human molecular genetics*, 23(11), pp. 2858–79.

Maiuolo, J. *et al.* (2016) 'Regulation of uric acid metabolism and excretion', *International Journal of Cardiology.* Elsevier B.V., 213, pp. 8–14.

Mankovskaya, I. N. *et al.* (2014) 'The effect of uridine on the endurance of animals with different resistance to physical stress: The role of mitochondrial ATP-dependent potassium channel', *Biophysics.* Pleiades Publishing, 59(5), pp. 764–767.

Marcinkiewicz, J. *et al.* (1998) 'Taurine chloramine down-regulates the generation of murine neutrophil inflammatory mediators', *Immunopharmacology*, 40(1), pp. 27–38.

Marcoff, L. and Thompson, P. D. (2007) 'The Role of Coenzyme Q10 in Statin-Associated Myopathy', *Journal of the American College of Cardiology*, 49(23), pp. 2231–2237.

Marcoux, F. W., Beal, M. F. and Choi, D. W. (2002) *CNS Neuroprotection.* Springer Science & Business Media.

Margittai, E. *et al.* (2005) 'Scurvy Leads to Endoplasmic Reticulum Stress and Apoptosis in the Liver of Guinea Pigs', *J. Nutr.*, 135(11), pp. 2530–2534.

Marras, C. and Saunders-Pullman, R. (2014) 'The complexities of hormonal influences and risk of Parkinson's disease.', *Movement disorders : official journal of the Movement Disorder Society*, 29(7), pp. 845–8.

Martin, W. F. and Mentel, M. (2010) 'Origin of Mitochondria', *Nature Education*, 3(9), p. 58.

Marwarha, G. *et al.* (2011) 'The oxysterol 27-hydroxycholesterol regulates α-synuclein and tyrosine hydroxylase expression levels in human neuroblastoma cells through modulation of liver X receptors and estrogen receptors--relevance to Parkinson's disease.', *Journal of neurochemistry*, 119(5), pp. 1119–36.

Masino, S. A. *et al.* (2016) 'Can Ketones Help Rescue Brain Fuel Supply in Later Life? Implications for Cognitive Health during Aging and the Treatment of Alzheimer's Disease', *Frontiers in molecular neuroscience.* Frontiers Media SA, 9(July), pp. 1–21.

Mattson, M. P. and Liu, D. (2002) 'Energetics and oxidative stress in synaptic plasticity and neurodegenerative disorders.', *Neuromolecular medicine*, 2(2), pp. 215–31.

Mazzio, E. *et al.* (2013) 'High throughput screening to identify natural human monoamine oxidase B inhibitors.', *Phytotherapy research : PTR*, 27(6), pp. 818–28.

Mcbean, G. J. (2012) 'Astrocytes and the regulation of cerebral cysteine/cystine redox potential: implications for cysteine neurotoxicity', pp. 135–153.

McCarty, M. F. (2013) 'Nutraceutical strategies for ameliorating the toxic effects of alcohol.', *Medical hypotheses*, pp. 456–62.

McColl, B. W. *et al.* (2010) 'Increased brain microvascular MMP-9 and incidence of haemorrhagic transformation in obese mice after experimental stroke.', *Journal of cerebral blood flow and metabolism : official journal of the International Society of Cerebral Blood Flow and Metabolism*, 30(2), pp. 267–72.

McCormack, P. L. (2014) 'Rasagiline: A Review of Its Use in the Treatment of Idiopathic Parkinson's Disease', *CNS Drugs*, 28(11), pp. 1083–1097.

McMillan, G. (2005) 'Is electric arc welding linked to manganism or Parkinson's disease?', *Toxicological reviews*, 24(4), pp. 237–57.

Medlock, A. E. *et al.* (2009) 'Product release rather than chelation determines metal specificity for ferrochelatase.', *Journal of molecular biology*, 393(2), pp. 308–19.

Mehran S M, M. and B, G. (2013) 'Simultaneous determination of levodopa and carbidopa from fava bean, green peas and green beans by high performance liquid gas chromatography.', *Journal of clinical and diagnostic research : JCDR*, 7(6), pp. 1004–7.

Meiser, J., Weindl, D. and Hiller, K. (2013a) 'Complexity of dopamine metabolism', *Cell Communication and Signaling*, pp. 1–18.

Meiser, J., Weindl, D. and Hiller, K. (2013b) 'Complexity of dopamine metabolism', *Cell Communication and Signaling*, 11(34), pp. 1–18.

Menendez, J. a *et al.* (2009) 'Fatty acid synthase: association with insulin resistance, type 2 diabetes, and cancer.', *Clinical chemistry*, 55(3), pp. 425–38.

Mercado, G., Valdés, P. and Hetz, C. (2013) 'An ERcentric view of Parkinson's disease.', *Trends in molecular medicine*, 19(3), pp. 165–75. doi: 10.1016/j.molmed.2012.12.005.

Micheli, F. E. and LeWitt, P. A. (eds) (2014) *Chorea*. London: Springer London.

Miller, R. L. *et al.* (2009) 'Oxidative and inflammatory pathways in Parkinson's disease.', *Neurochemical research*, 34(1), pp. 55–65.

MISSALE, C. *et al.* (1998) 'Dopamine Receptors: From Structure to Function', *Physiol Rev*, 78(1), pp. 189–225.

Miyake, Y. *et al.* (2010) 'Dietary fat intake and risk of Parkinson's disease: a case-control study in Japan.', *Journal of the neurological sciences*, 288(1–2), pp. 117–22.

Moccia, M. *et al.* (2014) 'Is serum uric acid related to non-motor symptoms in de-novo Parkinson's disease patients?', *Parkinsonism & related disorders*. Elsevier, 20(7), pp. 772–5.

Moccia, M. *et al.* (2015) 'Uric acid relates to dopamine transporter availability in Parkinson's disease', *Acta Neurologica Scandinavica*, 131(2), pp. 127–131.

Moloney, T. C. *et al.* (2014) 'Heat shock protein 70 reduces α-synuclein-induced predegenerative neuronal dystrophy in the α-synuclein viral gene transfer rat model of Parkinson's disease.', *CNS neuroscience & therapeutics*, 20(1), pp. 50–8.

Mosharov, E. V, Borgkvist, A. and Sulzer, D. (2015) 'Presynaptic effects of levodopa and their possible role in dyskinesia.', *Movement disorders : official journal of the Movement Disorder Society*. NIH Public Access, 30(1), pp. 45–53.

Muhamad Noor Alfarizal Kamarudin, H. A. K. (2014) 'Protective effects of (R)-(+)-a-lipoic acid against MPP+-stimulated microglia cells and toxicity in dopaminergic SH-SY5Y cells through PI3K-Akt/GSK-3b pathway', in.

Müller, C. P. *et al.* (2014) 'Brain membrane lipids in major depression and anxiety disorders.', *Biochimica et biophysica acta*.

Müller, T. (2009) 'Possible treatment concepts for the levodopa-related hyperhomocysteinemia.', *Cardiovascular psychiatry and neurology*, 2009, p. 969752.

Musgrove, R. E. J., King, A. E. and Dickson, T. C. (2011) 'Neuroprotective upregulation of endogenous α-synuclein precedes ubiquitination in cultured dopaminergic neurons.', *Neurotoxicity research*, 19(4), pp. 592–602.

Nagasawa, K. *et al.* (2005) 'Transport mechanism for aluminum citrate at the blood-brain barrier: kinetic evidence implies involvement of system Xc- in immortalized rat brain endothelial cells.', *Toxicology letters*, 155(2), pp. 289–96.

Nakashima, Y. *et al.* (2014) 'Preventive effects of Chlorella on skeletal muscle atrophy in muscle-specific mitochondrial aldehyde dehydrogenase 2 activity-deficient mice.', *BMC complementary and alternative medicine*, 14, p. 390.

Neher, J. J. et al. (2013) 'Phagocytosis executes delayed neuronal death after focal brain ischemia.', *Proceedings of the National Academy of Sciences of the United States of America*, 110(43), pp. E4098-107.

Nickolai, B. and Kiss, C. (2016) '[Nutritional therapy of gout]', *Ther Umsch*, 73(3), pp. 153–158.

Nolan, Y. M., Sullivan, A. M. and Toulouse, A. (2013) 'Parkinson's disease in the nuclear age of neuroinflammation.', *Trends in molecular medicine*, 19(3), pp. 187–96.

Nunnari, J. and Suomalainen, A. (2012) 'Mitochondria: in sickness and in health.', *Cell*. Elsevier Inc., 148(6), pp. 1145–59.

O'Keefe, J. H. et al. (2013) 'Effects of Habitual Coffee Consumption on Cardiometabolic Disease, Cardiovascular Health, and All-Cause Mortality', *Journal of the American College of Cardiology*. Journal of the American College of Cardiology, 62(12), pp. 1043–1051.

Ouzzine, M. et al. (2014) 'The UDP-glucuronosyltransferases of the blood-brain barrier: their role in drug metabolism and detoxication', *Frontiers in Cellular Neuroscience*. Frontiers, 8 (October), p. 349.

de Pablos, R. M. et al. (2014) 'Chronic stress enhances microglia activation and exacerbates death of nigral dopaminergic neurons under conditions of inflammation.', *Journal of neuroinflammation*, 11(1), p. 34.

Pais, T. F. et al. (2013) 'The NAD-dependent deacetylase sirtuin 2 is a suppressor of microglial activation and brain inflammation.', *The EMBO journal*, 32(19), pp. 2603–16.

Pakpoor, J. et al. (2015) 'Clinical associations between gout and multiple sclerosis, Parkinson's disease and motor neuron disease: record-linkage studies.', *BMC neurology*. BioMed Central, 15(1), p. 16.

Pan, T. et al. (2005) 'Valproic acid-mediated Hsp70 induction and anti-apoptotic neuroprotection in SH-SY5Y cells.', *FEBS letters*. Elsevier, 579(30), pp. 6716–20.

Pan, T. et al. (2008) 'The role of autophagy-lysosome pathway in neurodegeneration associated with Parkinson's disease.', *Brain : a journal of neurology*, 131(Pt 8), pp. 1969–78.

Paoli, A. et al. (2014) 'Ketogenic diet in neuromuscular and neurodegenerative diseases', *BioMed Research International*. Hindawi Publishing Corporation, p. 474296.

Perier, C. and Vila, M. (2012) 'Mitochondrial biology and Parkinson's disease.', *Cold Spring Harbor perspectives in medicine*. Cold Spring Harbor Laboratory Press, 4(1–19), p. a009332.

Peter Guengerich, F. *et al.* (2003) 'Cytochrome P450 1B1: a target for inhibition in anticarcinogenesis strategies', *Mutation Research/Fundamental and Molecular Mechanisms of Mutagenesis*, 523–524, pp. 173–182.

Phan, C. W. *et al.* (2015) 'Uridine from pleurotus giganteus and its neurite outgrowth stimulatory effects with underlying mechanism', *PLoS ONE*. Edited by F. Gallyas. Public Library of Science, 10(11), p. e0143004.

Pieczenik, S. R. and Neustadt, J. (2007) 'Mitochondrial dysfunction and molecular pathways of disease.', *Experimental and molecular pathology*, 83(1), pp. 84–92.

Pinckaers, P. J. M. *et al.* (2016) 'Ketone Bodies and Exercise Performance: The Next Magic Bullet or Merely Hype?', *Sports Medicine*, 18 July, pp. 1–9.

Politis, M. *et al.* (2014) 'Serotonergic mechanisms responsible for levodopa-induced dyskinesias in Parkinson's disease patients.', *The Journal of clinical investigation*. American Society for Clinical Investigation, 124(3), pp. 1340–9.

Porcheray, F. *et al.* (2006) 'Glutamate metabolism in HIV-infected macrophages: implications for the CNS.', *American journal of physiology. Cell physiology*, 291(4), pp. C618-26.

Purves, D. *et al.* (2001) 'Projections to the Basal Ganglia', in *Neuroscience 2nd Edition*. Sinauer Associates.

Rajendram, R., Preedy, V. R. and Patel, V. B. (eds) (2015) *Glutamine in Clinical Nutrition*. New York, NY: Springer New York.

Rajput, A. H. *et al.* (1997) 'Is levodopa toxic to human substantia nigra?', *Movement disorders : official journal of the Movement Disorder Society*, 12(5), pp. 634–8.

Rajput, A. H. (2001) 'Levodopa prolongs life expectancy and is non-toxic to substantia nigra', *Parkinsonism & Related Disorders*, 8(2), pp. 95–100.

Rantham Prabhakara, J. P. *et al.* (2008) 'Differential effects of 24-hydroxycholesterol and 27-hydroxycholesterol on tyrosine hydroxylase and alpha-synuclein in human neuroblastoma SH-SY5Y cells.', *Journal of neurochemistry*, 107(6), pp. 1722–9.

Rehnmark, A. and Strömberg, I. (2012) 'Antioxidant-Enriched Diet Affects Early Microglia Accumulation and Promotes Regeneration of the Striatal Dopamine System After a 6-Hydroxidopamine-Induced Lesion in a Rat', *Journal of Experimental Neuroscience*, 6, p. 21.

Rezai-Zadeh, K. *et al.* (2008) 'Apigenin and luteolin modulate microglial activation via inhibition of STAT1-induced CD40 expression.', *Journal of neuroinflammation*, 5, p. 41.

Rojo, A. I. *et al.* (2010) 'Nrf2 regulates microglial dynamics and neuroinflammation in experimental Parkinson's disease.', *Glia*, 58(5), pp. 588–98.

Rojo, A. I. *et al.* (2014) 'Redox Control of Microglial Function: Molecular Mechanisms and Functional Significance.', *Antioxidants & redox signaling*, pp. 1–37.

Rosell, A. *et al.* (2008) 'MMP-9-positive neutrophil infiltration is associated to blood-brain barrier breakdown and basal lamina type IV collagen degradation during hemorrhagic transformation after human ischemic stroke.', *Stroke; a journal of cerebral circulation*, 39(4), pp. 1121–6.

Rostovtseva, T. K. *et al.* (2015) 'α-Synuclein Shows High Affinity Interaction with Voltage-dependent Anion Channel, Suggesting Mechanisms of Mitochondrial Regulation and Toxicity in Parkinson Disease.', *The Journal of biological chemistry*, 290(30), pp. 18467–77.

Rouse, M., Younès, A. and Egan, J. M. (2014) 'Resveratrol and curcumin enhance pancreatic β-cell function by inhibiting phosphodiesterase activity.', *The Journal of endocrinology*, 223(2), pp. 107–17.

Royer, M.-C. *et al.* (2009) '7-ketocholesterol incorporation into sphingolipid/cholesterol-enriched (lipid raft) domains is impaired by vitamin E: a specific role for alpha-tocopherol with consequences on cell death.', *The Journal of biological chemistry*, 284(23), pp. 15826–34.

Rozema, D. and Gellman, S. H. (1996) 'Artificial chaperone-assisted refolding of denatured-reduced lysozyme: modulation of the competition between renaturation and aggregation.', *Biochemistry*, 35(49), pp. 15760–71.

Rugbjerg, K. *et al.* (2012) 'Malignant melanoma, breast cancer and other cancers in patients with Parkinson's disease.', *International journal of cancer. Journal international du cancer*, 131(8), pp. 1904–11.

Rutkevich, L. a and Williams, D. B. (2012) 'Vitamin K epoxide reductase contributes to protein disulfide formation and redox homeostasis within the endoplasmic reticulum.', *Molecular biology of the cell*, 23(11), pp. 2017–27.

Ryu, J. *et al.* (2010) 'Proteomic analysis of osteoclast lipid rafts: the role of the integrity of lipid rafts on V-ATPase activity in osteoclasts.', *Journal of bone and mineral metabolism*, 28(4), pp. 410–7.

Sahara, S. and Yamashima, T. (2010) 'Calpain-mediated Hsp70.1 cleavage in hippocampal CA1 neuronal death.', *Biochemical and biophysical research communications*, 393(4), pp. 806–11.

Sai, Y. *et al.* (2012) 'The Parkinson's Disease-related genes act in mitochondrial homeostasis', *Neuroscience & Biobehavioral Reviews*, 36(9), pp. 2304–2043.

Saligan, L. N. *et al.* (2013) 'Upregulation of α-synuclein during localized radiation therapy signals the association of cancer-related fatigue with the activation of inflammatory and neuroprotective pathways.', *Brain, behavior, and immunity*, 27(1), pp. 63–70.

Sampat, R. *et al.* (2016) 'Potential mechanisms for low uric acid in Parkinson disease', *Journal of Neural Transmission*. Springer Vienna, 123(4), pp. 365–370.

Sandur, S. K. *et al.* (2007) 'Role of pro-oxidants and antioxidants in the anti-inflammatory and apoptotic effects of curcumin (diferuloylmethane).', *Free radical biology & medicine*, 43(4), pp. 568–80.

Santiago, J. A. and Potashkin, J. A. (2015) 'Network-based metaanalysis identifies HNF4A and PTBP1 as longitudinally dynamic biomarkers for Parkinson's disease.', *Proceedings of the National Academy of Sciences of the United States of America*, 112(7), pp. 2257–62.

Santiago, J. a and Potashkin, J. a (2013) 'Shared dysregulated pathways lead to Parkinson's disease and diabetes.', *Trends in molecular medicine*. Elsevier Ltd, 19(3), pp. 176–86.

Sarbishegi, M., Mehraein, F. and Soleimani, M. (2014) 'Antioxidant role of oleuropein on midbrain and dopaminergic neurons of substantia nigra in aged rats.', *Iranian biomedical journal*, 18(1), pp. 16–22.

Schatz, I. J. *et al.* (2001) 'Cholesterol and all-cause mortality in elderly people from the Honolulu Heart Program: a cohort study', *The Lancet*, 358(9279), pp. 351–355. doi: 10.1016/S0140-6736(01)05553-2.

Schipper, H. M. et al. (2009) 'Heme oxygenase-1 and neurodegeneration: expanding frontiers of engagement.', *Journal of neurochemistry*, 110(2), pp. 469–85.

Schmidt, J. A. et al. (2013) 'Serum Uric Acid Concentrations in Meat Eaters, Fish Eaters, Vegetarians and Vegans: A Cross-Sectional Analysis in the EPIC-Oxford Cohort', *PLoS ONE*. Edited by O. Y. Gorlova, 8(2), p. e56339.

Schmitz, G. and Grandl, M. (2007) 'Role of redox regulation and lipid rafts in macrophages during Ox-LDL-mediated foam cell formation.', *Antioxidants & redox signaling*, 9(9), pp. 1499–518.

Schreibelt, G. et al. (2007) 'Reactive oxygen species alter brain endothelial tight junction dynamics via RhoA, PI3 kinase, and PKB signaling.', *FASEB journal : official publication of the Federation of American Societies for Experimental Biology*, 21(13), pp. 3666–76.

Schwarzschild, M. A. et al. (2014) 'Inosine to increase serum and cerebrospinal fluid urate in Parkinson disease: a randomized clinical trial.', *JAMA neurology*, 71(2), pp. 141–50.

Schwingshackl, L. and Hoffmann, G. (2014) 'Monounsaturated fatty acids, olive oil and health status: a systematic review and meta-analysis of cohort studies.', *Lipids in health and disease*, 13(1), p. 154.

Scoditti, E. et al. (2012) 'Mediterranean diet polyphenols reduce inflammatory angiogenesis through MMP-9 and COX-2 inhibition in human vascular endothelial cells: a potentially protective mechanism in atherosclerotic vascular disease and cancer.', *Archives of biochemistry and biophysics*, 527(2), pp. 81–9.

Seidl, S. E. et al. (2014) 'The emerging role of nutrition in Parkinson's disease.', *Frontiers in aging neuroscience*, 6(March), p. 36.

Seidl, S. E. and Potashkin, J. A. (2011) 'The promise of neuroprotective agents in Parkinson's disease.', *Frontiers in neurology*, 2, p. 68.

Serhan, C. N. (2014) 'Pro-resolving lipid mediators are leads for resolution physiology.', *Nature*, 510(7503), pp. 92–101.

Shaltiel-Karyo, R. et al. (2013) 'A blood-brain barrier (BBB) disrupter is also a potent α-synuclein (α-syn) aggregation inhibitor: a novel dual mechanism of mannitol for the treatment of Parkinson disease (PD).', *The Journal of biological chemistry*, 288(24), pp. 17579–88.

Sharma, A. *et al.* (1999) 'D4 dopamine receptor-mediated phospholipid methylation and its implications for mental illnesses such as schizophrenia.', *Molecular psychiatry*, 4(3), pp. 235–246.

Shichiri, M. *et al.* (2014) 'DHA concentration of red blood cells is inversely associated with markers of lipid peroxidation in men taking DHA supplement.', *Journal of clinical biochemistry and nutrition*, 55(3), pp. 196–202.

Simons, K. and Toomre, D. (2000) 'Lipid Rafts and Signal Transduction', *Nature Reviews Molecular Cell Biology*, 1(October), pp. 31–41.

Skocaj, M. *et al.* (2011) 'Titanium dioxide in our everyday life; is it safe?', *Radiology and oncology*, 45(4), pp. 227–47.

Song, C. *et al.* (2006) 'Omega-3 Fatty Acid Ethyl-Eicosapentaenoate Attenuates IL-1β-Induced Changes in Dopamine and Metabolites in the Shell of the Nucleus Accumbens: Involved with PLA2 Activity and Corticosterone Secretion', *Neuropsychopharmacology*, 32(3), pp. 736–744.

Srinivasan, V. *et al.* (2011) 'Melatonin in mitochondrial dysfunction and related disorders.', *International journal of Alzheimer's disease*, 2011, p. 326320.

Staubach, S. and Hanisch, F. (2011) 'Lipid rafts: signaling and sorting platforms of cells and their roles in cancer', *Expert Rev. Proteomics*, 8(2), pp. 263–277.

Steneberg, P. *et al.* (2013) 'The type 2 diabetes-associated gene ide is required for insulin secretion and suppression of α-synuclein levels in β-cells.', *Diabetes*, 62(6), pp. 2004–14.

Strushkevich, N. *et al.* (2011) 'Structural basis for pregnenolone biosynthesis by the mitochondrial monooxygenase system.', *Proceedings of the National Academy of Sciences of the United States of America*, 108(25), pp. 10139–43.

Stulnig, T. M. (1998) 'Polyunsaturated Fatty Acids Inhibit T Cell Signal Transduction by Modification of Detergent-insoluble Membrane Domains', *The Journal of Cell Biology*, 143(3), pp. 637–644.

Sun, A. Y. *et al.* (2010) 'Resveratrol as a therapeutic agent for neurodegenerative diseases.', *Molecular neurobiology*, 41(2–3), pp. 375–83.

Surh, Y.-J. (2012) 'Nrf2, an Essential Component of Cellular Stress Response, as a Potential Target of Hormetic Phytochemicals.', *Journal of Food and Drug Analysis,* 20(supplement 1), pp. 217–219.

Surh, Y.-J. and Kim, H.-J. (2010) 'Neurotoxic effects of tetrahydroisoquinolines and underlying mechanisms.', *Experimental neurobiology*, 19(2), pp. 63–70.

Surmeier, D. J. et al. (2011) 'The origins of oxidant stress in Parkinson's disease and therapeutic strategies.', *Antioxidants & redox signaling*. Mary Ann Liebert, Inc. 140 Huguenot Street, 3rd Floor New Rochelle, NY 10801 USA, 14(7), pp. 1289–301.

Swanson, J. . et al. (2000) 'Dopamine genes and ADHD', *Neuroscience & Biobehavioral Reviews*, 24(1), pp. 21–25.

Szabo, G. et al. (2007) 'TLR4, Ethanol, and Lipid Rafts: A New Mechanism of Ethanol Action with Implications for other Receptor-Mediated Effects', *The Journal of Immunology*. American Association of Immunologists, 178(3), pp. 1243–1249.

Takechi, R. et al. (2013) 'Nutraceutical agents with anti-inflammatory properties prevent dietary saturated-fat induced disturbances in blood-brain barrier function in wild-type mice.', *Journal of neuroinflammation*, 10, p. 73.

Takenouchi, T. et al. (2009) 'The role of the P2X7 receptor signaling pathway for the release of autolysosomes in microglial cells.', *Autophagy*, 5(5), pp. 723–4.

Tan, H. et al. (2012) 'Mood stabilizer lithium inhibits amphetamine-increased 4-hydroxynonenal-protein adducts in rat frontal cortex.', *The international journal of neuropsychopharmacology / official scientific journal of the Collegium Internationale Neuropsychopharmacologicum (CINP)*, 15(9), pp. 1275–85.

Tanabe, A. et al. (2014) 'A novel tyrosine kinase inhibitor AMN107 (nilotinib) normalizes striatal motor behaviors in a mouse model of Parkinson's disease.', *Frontiers in cellular neuroscience*. Frontiers, 8, p. 50.

Tanner, C. M. et al. (2011) 'Rotenone, paraquat, and Parkinson's disease.', *Environmental health perspectives*, 119(6), pp. 866–72.

Teismann, P. (2012) 'COX-2 in the neurodegenerative process of Parkinson's disease.', *BioFactors (Oxford, England)*, 38(6), pp. 395–7.

Teran-Garcia, M. et al. (2007) 'Polyunsaturated fatty acid suppression of fatty acid synthase (FASN): evidence for dietary modulation of NF-Y binding to the Fasn promoter by SREBP-1c.', *The Biochemical journal*, 402(3), pp. 591–600.

Theoharides, T. C. and Zhang, B. (2011) 'Neuro-inflammation, blood-brain barrier, seizures and autism.', *Journal of neuroinflammation*. BioMed Central Ltd, 8(1), p. 168.

Thomas, A. G. et al. (2014) 'Small molecule glutaminase inhibitors block glutamate release from stimulated microglia.', *Biochemical and biophysical research communications*, 443(1), pp. 32–6.

Thomas, B. (2009) 'Parkinson's disease: from molecular pathways in disease to therapeutic approaches.', *Antioxidants & redox signaling*, 11(9), pp. 2077–82.

Thomas, B. and Beal, M. F. (2007) 'Parkinson's disease.', *Human molecular genetics*, 16 Spec No(R2), pp. R183-94.

Trudler, D., Farfara, D. and Frenkel, D. (2010) 'Toll-like receptors expression and signaling in glia cells in neuro-amyloidogenic diseases: towards future therapeutic application.', *Mediators of inflammation*, 2010.

Tufekci, K. U. et al. (2011) 'The Nrf2/ARE Pathway: A Promising Target to Counteract Mitochondrial Dysfunction in Parkinson's Disease.', *Parkinson's disease*, 2011, p. 314082.

Turrens, J. F. (2003) 'Mitochondrial formation of reactive oxygen species', *The Journal of Physiology*, 552(2), pp. 335–344.

Ulluwishewa, D. et al. (2011) 'Regulation of tight junction permeability by intestinal bacteria and dietary components.', *The Journal of nutrition*, 141(5), pp. 769–76.

Via, M. (2012) 'The malnutrition of obesity: micronutrient deficiencies that promote diabetes.', *ISRN endocrinology*, 2012, p. 103472.

Viles, J. H. (2012) 'Metal ions and amyloid fiber formation in neurodegenerative diseases. Copper, zinc and iron in Alzheimer's, Parkinson's and prion diseases', *Coordination Chemistry Reviews*, 256(19–20), pp. 2271–2284.

Vitte, J. et al. (2004) 'Oxidative stress level in circulating neutrophils is linked to neurodegenerative diseases.', *Journal of clinical immunology*, 24(6), pp. 683–92.

Walker, F. R., Nilsson, M. and Jones, K. (2013) 'Acute and chronic stress-induced disturbances of microglial plasticity, phenotype and function.', *Current drug targets*, 14(11), pp. 1262–76.

Wallace, D. C., Fan, W. and Procaccio, V. (2010) 'Mitochondrial energetics and therapeutics.', *Annual review of pathology*, 5, pp. 297–348.

Wan, J. *et al.* (2007) 'Palmitoylated proteins: purification and identification.', *Nature protocols*. Nature Publishing Group, 2(7), pp. 1573–84.

Wang, J.-Y. *et al.* (2001) 'Vitamin D3 attenuates 6-hydroxydopamine-induced neurotoxicity in rats', *Brain Research*, 904(1), pp. 67–75.

Wang, L. *et al.* (2015) 'DHA inhibited AGEs-induced retinal microglia activation via suppression of the PPARγ/NFκB pathway and reduction of signal transducers in the AGEs/RAGE axis recruitment into lipid rafts.', *Neurochemical research*, 40(4), pp. 713–22.

Wang, X. *et al.* (2005) 'Genistein protects dopaminergic neurons by inhibiting microglial activation.', *Neuroreport*, 16(3), pp. 267–70.

Wasse, H. *et al.* (2011) '25-hydroxyvitamin D concentration is inversely associated with serum MMP-9 in a cross-sectional study of African American ESRD patients.', *BMC nephrology*, 12, p. 24.

Wei, C., Crane, B. and Stuehr, D. (2003) 'Tetrahydrobiopterin radical enzymology', *Chemical reviews*, 103, pp. 2635–2383.

Weise, C. *et al.* (2011) 'Inhibition of IgE production by docosahexaenoic acid is mediated by direct interference with STAT6 and NFκB pathway in human B cells.', *The Journal of nutritional biochemistry*, 22(3), pp. 269–75.

Wenzel, P. *et al.* (2007) 'Role of reduced lipoic acid in the redox regulation of mitochondrial aldehyde dehydrogenase (ALDH-2) activity. Implications for mitochondrial oxidative stress and nitrate tolerance.', *The Journal of biological chemistry*, 282(1), pp. 792–9.

Wilhelm, I., Fazakas, C. and Krizbai, I. A. (2011) 'In vitro models of the blood-brain barrier.', *Acta neurobiologiae experimentalis*, 71(1), pp. 113–28.

Wolf, A. M. *et al.* (2010) 'Astaxanthin protects mitochondrial redox state and functional integrity against oxidative stress.', *The Journal of nutritional biochemistry*, 21(5), pp. 381–9.

Wong, S. W. *et al.* (2009) 'Fatty Acids Modulate Toll-like Receptor 4 Activation through Regulation of Receptor Dimerization and Recruitment into Lipid Rafts in a Reactive Oxygen Species-dependent Manner', *Journal of Biological Chemistry*, 284(40), pp. 27384–27392.

Wright, R. O. and Baccarelli, A. (2007) 'Metals and Neurotoxicology', *J. Nutr.*, 137(12), pp. 2809–2813.

Wu, A. *et al.* (2015) 'Curcumin boosts DHA in the brain: Implications for the prevention of anxiety disorders.', *Biochimica et biophysica acta*, 1852(5), pp. 951–61.

Wu, J. *et al.* (2013) 'Neuroprotection by curcumin in ischemic brain injury involves the Akt/Nrf2 pathway.', *PloS one*, 8(3), p. e59843.

Wu, J. and Xie, H. (2014) 'Effects of titanium dioxide nanoparticles on α-synuclein aggregation and the ubiquitin-proteasome system in dopaminergic neurons.', *Artificial cells, nanomedicine, and biotechnology*. Informa Healthcare New York, pp. 1–5.

Wurtman, R. J., Cansev, M. and Ulus, I. H. (2009) 'Synapse formation is enhanced by oral administration of uridine and DHA, the circulating precursors of brain phosphatides', *Journal of Nutrition, Health and Aging*. Springer-Verlag, 13(3), pp. 189–197.

Xiao, H. (2015) 'Mechanisms Underlying Chemopreventive Effects of Flavonoids via Multiple Signaling Nodes within Nrf2-ARE and AhR-XRE Gene Regulatory Networks', *Current Chemical Biology*, 7(2).

Xie, L. *et al.* (2013) 'Sleep drives metabolite clearance from the adult brain.', *Science (New York, N.Y.)*, 342(6156), pp. 373–7.

Xilouri, M., Brekk, O. R. and Stefanis, L. (2013) 'α-Synuclein and protein degradation systems: a reciprocal relationship.', *Molecular neurobiology*, 47(2), pp. 537–51.

Xu, J. and Drew, P. (2006) '9- Cis-retinoic acid suppresses inflammatory responses of microglia and astrocytes', *Journal of neuroimmunology*, 171, pp. 135–144.

Xu, M.-X. *et al.* (2013) 'Resolvin D1, an endogenous lipid mediator for inactivation of inflammation-related signaling pathways in microglial cells, prevents lipopolysaccharide-induced inflammatory responses.', *CNS neuroscience & therapeutics*, 19(4), pp. 235–43.

Yamaguchi, T. *et al.* (1983) 'Effects of tyrosine administration on serum biopterin in normal controls and patients with Parkinson's disease', *Science*. American Association for the Advancement of Science, 219(4580), pp. 75–77.

Yamashima, T. *et al.* (2001) 'Neuroprotective effects of pyridoxal phosphate and pyridoxal against ischemia in monkeys.', *Nutritional neuroscience*, 4(5), pp. 389–97.

Yamashima, T. (2012) 'Hsp70.1 and related lysosomal factors for necrotic neuronal death.', *Journal of neurochemistry*, 120(4), pp. 477–94.

Yang, Y. *et al.* (2014) 'Characterization of food-grade titanium dioxide: the presence of nanosized particles.', *Environmental science & technology*, 48(11), pp. 6391–400.

Yang, Y. and Rosenberg, G. a (2011) 'Blood-brain barrier breakdown in acute and chronic cerebrovascular disease.', *Stroke; a journal of cerebral circulation*, 42(11), pp. 3323–8.

Yao, J. *et al.* (2003) 'Catechol Estrogen 4-Hydroxyequilenin Is a Substrate and an Inhibitor of Catechol- O -Methyltransferase', *Chemical Research in Toxicology*. American Chemical Society, 16(5), pp. 668–675.

Yao, Y. and Tsirka, S. E. (2014) 'Monocyte chemoattractant protein-1 and the blood-brain barrier.', *Cellular and molecular life sciences : CMLS*, 71(4), pp. 683–97.

Yokota, T. *et al.* (2001) 'Delayed-onset ataxia in mice lacking alpha -tocopherol transfer protein: model for neuronal degeneration caused by chronic oxidative stress.', *Proceedings of the National Academy of Sciences of the United States of America*. National Academy of Sciences, 98(26), pp. 15185–90.

Yorimitsu, T. and Klionsky, D. J. (2005) 'Autophagy: molecular machinery for self-eating.', *Cell death and differentiation*, 12 Suppl 2(S2), pp. 1542–52.

Youdim, M. B., Gross, A. and Finberg, J. P. (2001) 'Rasagiline [N-propargyl-1R(+)-aminoindan], a selective and potent inhibitor of mitochondrial monoamine oxidase B.', *British journal of pharmacology*, 132(2), pp. 500–6.

Zahid, M. *et al.* (2011) 'Formation of dopamine quinone-DNA adducts and their potential role in the etiology of Parkinson's disease.', *IUBMB life*, 63(12), pp. 1087–93.

Zecca, L. *et al.* (2001) 'Substantia nigra neuromelanin: structure, synthesis, and molecular behaviour.', *Molecular pathology : MP*. BMJ Group, 54(6), pp. 414–8.

Zhang, M., Picard-Deland, E. and Marette, A. (2013) 'Fish and marine omega-3 polyunsatured fatty acid consumption and incidence of type 2 diabetes: a systematic review and meta-analysis', *International journal of endocrinology*, 2013, pp. 20–22.

Zhang, Y. *et al.* (2013) 'The effect of alpha-synuclein overexpression on the process of cellular energy metabolism in transgenic mouse model', in *2013 ICME International Conference on Complex Medical Engineering*. IEEE, pp. 244–248.

Zhang, Y. *et al.* (2016) 'Decreased brain levels of vitamin B12 in aging, autism and schizophrenia', *PLoS ONE*. Edited by J. A. Bauer. Public Library of Science, 11(1), p. e0146797.

Zhao, L. *et al.* (2013) 'Early intervention with an estrogen receptor β-selective phytoestrogenic formulation prolongs survival, improves spatial recognition memory, and slows progression of amyloid pathology in a female mouse model of Alzheimer's disease.', *Journal of Alzheimer's disease : JAD*, 37(2), pp. 403–19.

Zhong, Z. *et al.* (2008) 'ALS-causing SOD1 mutants generate vascular changes prior to motor neuron degeneration.', *Nature neuroscience*. Nature Publishing Group, 11(4), pp. 420–2.

Zhou, M. *et al.* (2015) 'Neuronal death induced by misfolded prion protein is due to NAD^+ depletion and can be relieved in vitro and in vivo by NAD^+ replenishment.', *Brain : a journal of neurology*, 138(Pt 4), pp. 992–1008.

Zhu, B. (2002) 'Catechol-O-Methyltransferase (COMT)-Mediated Methylation Metabolism of Endogenous Bioactive Catechols and Modulation by Endobiotics and Xenobiotics: Importance in Pathophysiology and Pathogenesis', *Current Drug Metabolism*, 3(3), pp. 321–349.

Further reading

www.parkinsons.org.uk
Parkinson's UK

www.epda.eu.com
The European Parkinson's Disease Association

www.worldpdcoalition.org
The World Parkinson's Coalition

www.michaeljfox.org
The Michael J. Fox Foundation for Parkinson's Research

Everything You Need to Know about Parkinson's Disease
Lianna Marie (Create Space) 2015

Everything You Need to Know about Caregiving for Parkinson's Disease – Lianna Marie (Create Space) 2016

Lucky Man: A Memoir
Michael J. Fox (Ebury Press) 2003

Parkinson's Disease: A Complete Guide for Patients and Families
Weiner MD, William J., Shulman MD, Lisa M., et al. (John Hopkins Press) 2014

Parkinson's Disease: How to Optimise ON-OFF Periods during L-dopa Therapy – Dr Geoffrey Leader, Lucille Leader, Foreword: Professor Leslie Findley (Denor Press) 2019

Parkinson's Disease: Reducing Symptoms with Nutrition and Drugs – Dr Geoffrey Leader, Lucille Leader, Foreword: Professor Leslie Findley (Denor Press) 2018

Index

A

α-linolenic acid (ALA) 30, 33
α-lipoic acid 4, 19, 22, 41, 48, 66
α-synuclein vii, 2, 4, 10-16, 19-22, 24, 30, 32, 33, 35-38, 46, 47, 54, 55, 57-62, 66, 75-77
α-tocopherol 39
AADC (aromatic L-amino acid decarboxylase) 5, 8, 72, 73
acetaldehyde 53
acetoacetate 80
acetone 80
acetylsalicylic acid 22
acidosis 81
actin 69
adduct 26, 41, 42, 43, 63
adenosine 13, 17, 55
adenosine A2A and A2B receptors 13, 55
adenosine diphosphate (ADP) 17
adenosine triphosphate (ATP) 1, 15, 17, 19, 20, 22, 58, 60, 68, 78, 81
adrenaline 5
aggregates 10, 12, 15, 16, 19, 21, 62
alcohol 39, 44, 53, 54, 56, 79
aldehyde vii, 2, 7, 12, 44, 49, 53, 63
ALDH (aldehyde dehydrogenase) 2-4, 49, 63
algae 4, 64
allergy 37, 53
ALA (α-linolenic acid) 30, 33
aluminium 22, 51, 52, 56, 58, 60, 61, 78
aluminosilicate 11
Alzheimer's disease 1, 10, 21, 22, 36, 38, 57, 62, 66, 76, 80, 86
amino acid 5, 6, 8-10, 24, 25, 42, 48, 53, 74, 83
ammonia 2
amphetamine 2, 3
amylin (IAPP) 65, 66
amyloid precursor protein (APP) 38
amyloid protein 66
amyloid-β 21, 22, 38, 57, 65, 66
anaemia 9
anaerobic 17, 19
anti-ageing 64
anti-inflammatory 30, 31, 37, 39
antioxidant 4, 6, 19, 20, 26, 32, 42-44, 48, 49, 63, 66, 78
antioxidant response element (ARE) 42, 19
apigenin 49
apoptosis 19, 21, 24, 30, 32, 34, 36, 46, 59, 76

arachidonic acid (AA) 32
aromatic 25, 27, 28
aromatic L-amino acid decarboxylase (AADC) 5, 6, 8, 9, 72, 73
arsenic 58
aryl hydrocarbon receptor 27
asbestos 78
ascorbate 8, 19, 24, 55
Aspirin (acetylsalicylic acid) 22
astaxanthin 19
astrocyte 57
atherosclerosis 38
ATP (adenosine triphosphate) 1, 15, 17, 19, 20, 22, 58, 60, 68, 78, 81
ATP13A2 15, 16
ATPase 15
autophagic 14, 15
autophagosome 14, 15
autophagy 14, 15
autophagy-lysosome pathway (ALP) vii, 12, 14
autoxidation 1, 8
avocado 36
axon 1, 18, 69, 86
ayurvedic medicine 9

B

β-oxidation 80
β-sitosterol 36
bacteria 11, 31, 54
barberry 4
basal ganglia 1, 73, 83, 74
bauxite 60
Bax (Bcl-2-associated X protein) 34, 76
B-cells 37
BDNF (brain-derived neurotrophic factor) 50
benfotiamine 50
benserazide 8, 9, 55
benzene 25, 26, 42
berberine 4
Berberis vulgaris 4
berry anthocyanins 3
beta-hydroxybutyrate 80
Bifidobacterium infantis 54
bilberry 49
biogenesis 19, 42
bipolar disorder 63
bovine brain cortex 33
blueberry 49
Braak hypothesis vii, 10, 11
bradykinesia 1

broccoli 19
bromelain 49
buffer 23
butyrate 29

C

calpain 15
catechin 3, 27
catechol 25, 27, 41, 42, 43, 44
catechol oestrogen 26, 41, 44
catechol quinones 41, 42
catecholaldehyde hypothesis vii, 3
catecholamine 5, 25, 41, 73
catechol-o-methyltransferase (COMT) 41
cathepsin 15, 16
cerebrospinal fluid 44
ceruloplasmin 61
chaperone-mediated autophagy 14
chaperone 15, 62, 64
chemokine 51
chlorella 4, 64
chlorophyll 22
cholesterol 23, 34-37, 39, 78
cholesterol efflux 36
choline 84, 86
chorea 71
chylomicrons 80
cinnamon 42
citrate 60
citric 60
CJD (Creutzfeldt-Jakob disease) 10
CNS (central nervous system) 27, 29, 31, 33, 35, 36, 38, 46, 49-51, 54, 65
cobalt 58
coconut 31
coenzyme Q10 (CoQ10) 19, 36, 42, 64
coffee 13, 55, 79
collagen 52, 53
COMT (catechol-o-methyltransferase) 41, 43, 44
conjugated equine oestrogen 43
constipation 81
copper 52, 58, 61, 66
CoQ10 (coenzyme Q10) 19, 36, 42, 64
cordyceps 85
corticotropin-releasing hormone (CRH) 53
COX (cyclooxygenase) 32
COX-1 (cyclooxygenase-1) 32
COX-2 (cyclooxygenase-2) 32, 42, 50, 59
Creutzfeldt-Jakob disease (CJD) 10, 11, 62

crowberry 49
cruciferous 42
curcumin 3, 12, 27, 30, 32, 43, 49, 67
cyclooxygenase (COX) 32
cyclooxygenase-2 (COX-2) 42, 50
CYP1B1 27, 42
CYP2E1 53
cysteine 16, 19, 34, 42, 48
cystine 48
cytokine 30, 31, 33, 35, 37, 46, 47, 49-51, 53, 59, 65
cytoskeletal track 18, 68
cytoskeleton 68

D

daidzein 36
deacetylase 47
decarboxylase inhibitor 6, 55
delta 5-desaturaturation 32
demethylation 13
denatured egg white 62
dendrite 69, 84
dephosphorylate 12
depurinating DNA adducts 41, 43
detoxification 3, 42, 53, 58, 85
DHA (docosahexaenoic acid) 4, 13, 30-33, 37, 38, 84, 86
diabetes 33, 43, 65-67, 75, 81
diamine oxidase 55, 56
diarrhoea 81
diindolylmethane 49
dioxin 27
DJ-1 38, 65, 75
DNA 26, 40-43, 78
docosahexaenoic acid (DHA) 30, 37
DOPAC 2
DOPAL vii, 2, 3, 7, 12, 31, 44, 45, 49, 53, 63
dopamine quinone 1, 19, 41, 44, 58
dopaminergic 1, 3-6, 13, 14, 20, 30, 32, 34, 36, 38, 46-51, 60, 66, 70-72, 76, 78, 81, 83, 84
dyskinesia 30, 71, 72
dystonia 71

E

EGCG (epigallocatechin-3-gallate) 12, 27, 42
EHT (eicosanoyl-5-hydroxytryptamide) 13
electron 17, 19, 64
electron transport chain (ECT) 1, 17-19, 21, 63, 67, 81, 85
endocrine 5, 26
endoplasmic reticulum (ER) vii, 12, 23, 35, 37, 59

endothelial 34, 51, 52, 54, 55
eNOS 34
enteric 11
EPA (eicosapentaenoic acid) 30, 32
epigallocatechin 12, 27
epigallocatechin-3-gallate (EGCG) 12, 27, 42
epilepsy 63, 80, 81
epinephrine 5
epithelium 54
equine 43
equol 36
ER (endoplasmic reticulum) vii, 12, 23, 35, 37, 59
ETC (electron transport chain) 1, 17-19, 21, 63, 67, 81, 85
eukaryotes 17
evolution 17, 60, 78
excitotoxic 48
excitotoxicity 15, 47, 51, 59, 76
excitotoxin 31, 47
exercise 50, 60, 86
extra-virgin olive oil 34

F

F-actin 84
familial Parkinson's disease 65, 75, 76
fatigue 18, 21
fats 29, 54, 80, 81
fatty acid 24, 29, 30, 31, 32, 37, 80, 84
fatty acid synthase (FASN) 33, 65
fatty acyl chain 13, 33
fatty microdomains 37
FDA (Federal Drug Administration - USA) 33
Fenton reaction 58
ferrochelatase 22
fibril 10, 12
folate 43
folic acid 86
freezing 70

G

gait 1
gastrointestinal 5, 10, 11, 47
GDNF (glial cell line-derived neurotrophic factor) 50
genes 65, 75, 84
genistein 36, 40
genotoxic 26, 27, 41, 44
giant oyster mushroom (Pleurotus giganteus) 84
ginseng 40, 49
ginsenoside Rg1 40

glia 57
gliadin 54
glial 39, 47, 50, 51, 57
glucagon 65
glucose 17, 33, 65, 66, 73, 81
glutamate 31, 47, 48, 59, 76, 77
glutaminase 47
glutamine 48
glutathione 8, 19, 24, 30, 41, 42, 48, 49, 81
gluten 54, 56
glycated protein (AGE) 37
glycated haemoglobin 66
glycine 48
glymphatic system viii, 57
gout 78, 79, 81
grapes 12, 42

H

haeme 17, 21, 22, 44
haemoglobin 66
haemolytic anaemia 9
heat-shock protein 62-64
high-carbohydrate diet 33, 65
high-fat diet 31
histamine 53, 55, 56, 73
histidine 55, 73
HMG-CoA reductase 23, 35
HNF4A (Hepatocyte nuclear factor 4 alpha) 75
HO-1 (haeme oxygenase-1) 22, 45
homocysteine 43, 44
hormone/hormones 5, 17, 20, 53, 66, 70
Hsp70 (heat-shock protein 70) 15, 63
Huntingdon's disease 10, 36, 62
hydrocarbon 25-27, 42, 85
hydrogen 17
hydrogen peroxide 1, 2, 8, 43, 46, 55
hydrophilic 35
hydrophobic 10
hydroxyl radical 8, 55, 58
hyperacetylation 47
hyperforin 49
hyperlipidaemia 81
hyperprolactinaemia 5
hypertension 78

I

ibuprofen 47
IgE 37
immobilisation stress 70

immune 39, 46, 51, 53
immune system vii, viii, 17, 31, 37
immunoglobulin 37, 53
inflammasome 78
iNOS (inducible nitric oxide synthase) 34, 42, 48, 50, 59
inosine 79
insulin 65, 66, 75, 81
insulin-degrading enzyme 30, 66
insulin resistance viii, 33, 43, 54, 65, 66
interleukin 1 51
intermembrane space 17
intestinal 11, 54, 72
islet amyloid polypeptide (IAPP or amylin) 65, 66

K

kaempferol 49
ketoacidosis 81, 82
ketogenic diet 34, 80, 81
ketone 80-82
ketosis 81, 82
kidney 5, 64, 78-81
kinesin protein motor 18, 68
kynurenine pathway 9

L

L. plantarum 54
L-DOPA (L-3,4-dihydroxyphenylalanine) 1, 3, 5-9, 44, 55, 56, 71-74
laurate 29, 31, 33, 65
LCFA (long-chain fatty acid) 80
leptin 43
leucine-rich repeat kinase 2 (LRRK2) 38, 75
levodopa 6, 43, 44
Lewy bodies and neurites vii, 10, 21, 58
lipoic acid 4, 19, 22, 41, 48, 66
lion's mane mushroom 24, 85
lipid 3, 13, 14, 23, 24, 29-32, 34-40, 49, 53, 55, 63, 70
lipid raft vii, viii, 31, 32, 33, 36-39, 49, 53
lipid peroxide 3, 32, 39, 40, 63, 70
lipid hydroperoxides 55
lipidation 34
lipogenic state 33, 65
lipophilic 35
lipopolysaccharide (LPS) 31
lithium 63, 64
liver 80
long-chain saturated fatty acid 34, 38
LRRK2 (leucine-rich repeat kinase 2) 38, 75
luteolin 3, 49

lycopene 43, 49
lymphatic 57, 80
lysosome vii, 12, 14-16

M

macroautophagy 14
macrophage 37, 38, 46, 53
magnesium 19, 43, 58, 60, 66, 81
malignant melanoma 41
MAM (mitochondria-associated ER membrane) vii, 24, 36, 38
MAM hypothesis vii, 36
manganese 22, 47-49, 52, 58, 59
manganism 47, 59
mannitol 54, 55
MAO (monoamine oxidase) 2-4, 31, 40, 59
MAO-B 4, 31
MAO-inhibition 3
MCP1 (Monocyte chemoattractant protein-1) 51
melanin 83
melatonin 20, 41
menopause 40
mercury 22, 58
metalloproteinase (MMP) 52, 53, 55, 56
methyl donor 43, 44
methylation 12, 41, 43
microautophagy 14
microglia viii, 27, 30, 31, 33, 37, 38, 46-51, 59, 60
microglial activation viii, 13, 32, 46-50, 70
microgliosis 46
microtubule 68, 69
misfolding vii, viii, 10-12, 20, 24, 30, 54, 57, 62, 64-66, 86
mitochondria 12, 15, 17-21, 23, 24, 34, 37, 59, 68, 76, 80, 81, 85
mitochondria-associated ER membrane (MAM) vii, 24, 36, 38
mitochondrial biogenesis 42
mitochondrion 18, 21, 23
mitophagy 76
MMP (metalloproteinase) 52, 53, 55, 56
monoamine oxidase (MAO) 2-4, 31, 40, 59
monocyte 51, 53, 55
monounsaturated fatty acid (MUFA) 29, 34
motile 18
motor 4, 5, 10, 76-78, 83, 84
motor neuron 64
motor neurone disease 10, 52, 79
MPP+ (1-methyl-4-phenylpyridinium) 2
MPTP (1-methyl4-phenyl-1,2,3,6-tetrahydropyridine) 47, 85
mRNA (messenger ribonucleic acid) 75
mucuna pruriens 9
MUFA (monounsaturated fatty acid) 29, 34

multiple sclerosis 36, 55, 79
mushroom 24, 84-86
myeloid leukaemia 76
myricetin 12
myristate 29

N

NAC (N-acetylcysteine) 41, 42, 44, 48
NAD$^+$ (nicotinamide adenine dinucleotide - oxidised) 20
NADH (nicotinamide adenine dinucleotide - reduced) 8, 17, 78
nervous system vii, viii, 10, 26, 37, 40, 79, 83
neurite 10
neurite outgrowth 24, 85, 86
neurodegeneration vii, viii, 14, 22, 32, 38, 41, 43, 50, 57, 66, 68, 85
neuroinflammation viii, 13, 22, 30, 38, 39, 46, 50-52, 55, 62
neurological 21, 44, 46, 59
neuromelanin 46, 58, 70, 83
neuron vii, 1, 3, 18, 20, 23, 33, 34, 47, 68
neuroprotectin D1 (NPD1) 30
neuroprotection 34, 63, 80, 81
neurotoxic 7, 31, 41, 44, 46, 58, 59, 85
neurotoxicity 12, 44, 48, 58, 60, 63
neurotoxin 2, 45
neurotransmitter 5, 25, 58, 71, 73, 74
neurovascular unit 51
neutrophil 53
NF-kB 47
nicotinamide coenzymes 9
nigrostriatal 1, 70, 73, 83, 84
nitric oxide 19, 22, 29, 34, 46, 47, 49, 53, 59
nitrosylation 12
NMDA receptor 59
N-methylated tetrahydroisoquinoline 44
nNOS (neuronal nitric oxide synthase) 59
noradrenaline 5
norepinephrine 5
NPD1 (neuroprotectin D1) 30
NQO1 ((NAD(P)H:quinone acceptor oxidoreductase 1) 42
Nrf2 19, 32, 42-44, 49
NSAID (nonsteroidal anti-inflammatory drug) 47
nucelosides 84
nuceotides 84
nutmeg 54
nuts 36

O

obesity 33, 52, 65, 66
oestradiol 40
oestrogen 26-28, 36, 40-44

oleuropein 34
olfactory vii, 10
oligomer 10, 66
oligomerization 55
olive oil 34, 55
omega-3 polyunsaturated fatty acid 4, 30-33, 37, 49, 65
omega-6 polyunsaturated fatty acid 30, 32
oncology 76
organelle 14, 17, 18, 23, 24, 29, 68, 76
orthopaedic implant 59, 60
osteoclast 38
osteoporosis 38
oxidation 2, 12, 24, 40
oxidative stress 15, 19, 21, 22, 35, 42, 43, 47, 48, 50, 52, 53, 76
oxysterol 35, 36

P

P2X7 (purine receptor) 15
palmitate 29, 33, 34, 37, 38, 54, 65
palmitoylation 34, 38, 53
pancreatic β cell 38, 65-67
pantethine 4
paprika 54
paraquat 47
PARK9 gene (aka ATP13A2 gene) 15
parkin 38, 75-77
Parkinson, James 1
parkinsonism 15, 63
pattern recognition receptor 31
peak-dose dyskinesia 71, 72
peas 9
peroxidation 22
peroxynitrite 19, 46
pesticide 19, 47, 51, 63
petrochemical 25
phagocytosis 33
phenolic compounds 4, 32
phosphatide 84, 86
phosphatidic acid 16
phosphatidylcholine 16, 84
phosphatidylethanolamine 84
phosphatidylinositol 84
phosphatidylserine 33, 84
phospholipase D2 16
phospholipase A2 (PLA2) 32, 59
phospholipid 13, 16, 23, 32, 33, 39, 84-86
phosphorylation 12, 76
phytoestrogens 36, 40
PINK1 (PTEN-induced putative kinase 1) 75

PLA2 (phospholipase A2) 32, 50
plastoquinone 64
PLM (phospholipid methylation) 86
PLP (pyridoxal 5'-phosphate) 16, 73
polyphenol 12, 25-28, 30, 34, 40, 43, 44, 49, 55, 67
polyunsaturated fatty acid 13, 29-33, 37-39, 49, 65
post-translational modification 12, 23, 29, 38
potassium 66
PP2A (protein phosphatase 2A) 12, 13, 30
PPAR-γ (peroxisome proliferator-activated receptor gamma) 30
presynaptic dysregulation 71
prion protein 11, 20
proapoptotic protein 34, 76
probiotic bacteria 54
pro-oxidant 43
pro-resolving lipid mediators 30
prostaglandin E2 53
prostate cancer 41
protectin 30
protein folding 15, 23, 24, 59
protein misfolding 10, 30, 54, 62, 65
protoporphyrin 22
psoriasis 64
psychological stress 53, 56, 70
PTBP1 (polypyrimidine tract binding protein 1) 75
PUFA (polyunsaturated fatty acid) 13, 29-33, 37-39, 49, 65
pulses 79
purine 15, 78, 79, 85
putamen 3
pyridoxal 5'-phosphate (PLP) 16, 73
pyrimidine nucleoside 85

Q

quercetin 3, 19, 27, 40, 54, 55
quinone 41, 42, 44, 64
quinoprotein 7, 58
quinotyrosine 7

R

radiation 21
radical 8, 19, 52, 55, 58, 78
raft vii, viii, 31-33, 36-39, 49, 53
rasagiline 3, 4
redox-cycling 7
reishi mushroom 85
resolvin D1 (RvD1) 30
resveratrol 19, 27, 40-42, 49, 55, 64, 67
retinaldehyde dehydrogenase 1 49
retinoic acid 49, 50

riboflavin 24
RNA (ribonucleic acid) 78
RNS (reactive nitrogen species) 19
rotenone 2, 19, 47, 63
rutin 3

S

S-acylation 34
S-adenosylhomocysteine 43
salicylic acid 22
SAM (S-adenosylmethionine) 43, 44
saturated fat/fatty acids 29, 31, 33-35, 37, 38, 54, 65, 80
sauna 63
schizophrenia 5
seed vii, 10, 11
selegiline 3, 4
semen 85
serotonergic neurons 71, 72
serotonin 72, 73
sesame oil 32
sesamin 32
Shaking Palsy 1
silicilic acid 60
silicon-rich mineral water 60
SIRT1 64
SIRT2 47
sirtuin 47
skimmed milk 59
soy phospholipid 33, 36, 40
sperm 85
sphingolipids 37
sphingomyelin 34, 38, 84
spinal cord 46
sporadic Parkinson's disease 75
statin 35, 36
stearate 33, 65
steelworkers 59
sterol 23, 36
striatal 71, 72, 84
striatum 1, 76, 77, 83, 84
substantia nigra vii, 1, 10, 34, 42, 58, 59, 83
sulforaphane 42
sulphur 19, 43
sunscreen 59
superoxide 1, 8, 19, 46, 49, 52
superoxide dismutase 52, 55
synapse 1, 12, 18, 68, 84-86
synapsin-1 84
syntaxin-3 84

T

taurine 4, 19, 53, 67
T-cells 37
tea 12, 27, 42, 49, 54
TEER (transepithelial electrical resistance) 54
temperature 62, 63
tethering 34, 37
tetrahydrobiopterin 70
tetrahydroisoquinoline 44
tetrahydropapaveroline 44, 45
tetrahydropyridine 85
theaflavins 12
thiol 4, 42, 66
tiger milk mushroom 85
tight junction 51, 52, 54
titanium dioxide 47, 59, 60
titanium dioxide nanoparticles 60
TLR4 31
TLR (toll-like receptor) 31
TNF alpha 51
tocopherol 24, 39
toll-like receptor (TLR) 31
Tourette's syndrome 5
transepithelial electrical resistance (TEER) 54
tremor 1, 5, 13, 83
tricarboxylic cycle 17, 19
triglycerides 80
tryptophan 9
tubulin, α and β 68
turmeric 12, 19, 32, 67
tyrosine 5, 8, 25, 83
tyrosine hydroxylase 1, 5-8, 27, 36, 44, 58, 70
tyrosine kinase inhibition 76
type 2 diabetes viii, 33, 43. 65, 66, 81

U

ubiquinone (see CoQ10) 42
ubiquitin proteasome system (UPS) 12, 14, 76
ubiquitination 12, 76
UDP-glucuronosyl-transferase (UGT) 85
unfrying an egg 62
uric acid 78, 79
uricase 78
uridine 84-86
ursolic acid 3

V

valproic acid 63
VDAC (voltage-dependent anion channel) 21

vegan 79
vegetarian 79
vesicle 1-4, 2, 11, 31, 63, 71, 85
vesicular monoamine transporter 2 (VMAT2) 1, 3, 4, 31, 63
vitamin 8, 9, 16, 19, 22, 24, 32, 39, 42, 49, 50, 55, 65, 73, 86
vitamin B12 22, 43, 86
vitamin B6 8, 9, 16, 22, 43, 73, 86
VMAT2 (vesicular monoamine transporter 2) 1, 3, 4, 31, 63
volatile organic compound 25, 26

W

walnuts 12
wasabi 42
wheat 54, 56

X

xanthine oxidase 59
xenobiotic 27, 28, 85

Y

young-onset Parkinson's disease 76

Z

Zn-SOD (zinc superoxide dismutase) 55
zonulin 54

1,25-dihydroxyvitamin 50
24S-hydroxycholesterol 36
27-hydroxycholesterol 36
3-O-methyldopa 43
4-hydroxyestrone 26, 27
4-hydroxylation 41, 42

Printed in Great Britain
by Amazon